Services and Business Process Reengineering

The book series aims at bringing together valuable and novel scientific contributions that address the critical issues of software services and business processes reengineering, providing innovative ideas, methodologies, technologies and platforms that have an impact in this diverse and fast-changing research community in academia and industry.

The areas to be covered are

- Service Design
- Deployment of Services on Cloud and Edge Computing Platform
- Web Services
- IoT Services
- Requirements Engineering for Software Services
- Privacy in Software Services
- Business Process Management
- Business Process Redesign
- Software Design and Process Autonomy
- Security as a Service
- IoT Services and Privacy
- Business Analytics and Autonomic Software Management
- Service Reengineering
- Business Applications and Service Planning
- Policy Based Software Development
- Software Analysis and Verification
- Enterprise Architecture

The series serves as a qualified repository for collecting and promoting state-of-the art research trends in the broad area of software services and business processes reengineering in the context of enterprise scenarios. The series will include monographs, edited volumes and selected proceedings.

Alessandro Bernes • Shaira Thobani
Editors

Digitalisation in Health Care between New Technologies, Data and Research

Springer

Editors
Alessandro Bernes
Department of Economics
Ca' Foscari University of Venice
Venice, Italy

Shaira Thobani
Department of Law
University of Turin
Torino, Italy

ISSN 2524-5503 ISSN 2524-5511 (electronic)
Services and Business Process Reengineering
ISBN 978-981-95-6981-6 ISBN 978-981-95-6982-3 (eBook)
https://doi.org/10.1007/978-981-95-6982-3

This Springer imprint is published by the registered company Springer Nature Singapore Pte Ltd.
The registered company address is: 152 Beach Road, #21-01/04 Gateway East, Singapore 189721, Singapore

Preface

As the principal investigator of PRIN 2022 PNRR "Privacy-Aware Data Sharing model for Health data" (PADS4Health), I am particularly honoured to introduce and present this conference, together with my colleague Prof. Shaira Thobani, head of the research unit at the University of Turin.

I must say that this conference aims at being not only an occasion of interdisciplinary dialogue, but also an opportunity for interprofessional conversation, looking at the distinguished speakers who will take turns and whom I thank again sincerely.

In these few opening remarks, I would like to highlight some legal aspects of digital health (eHealth), a broad and all-encompassing term that includes telemedicine, medical robotics, processing of personal data in healthcare for both treatment and scientific research purposes, etc.

First of all, let me clarify the context in which our conference and, in general, our project are taking place.

The healthcare system has been profoundly revolutionised with the advent of the digital age. In the medical field, however, digitisation is much more than a technical process: on the one hand, it certainly involves new technologies and algorithms, including artificial intelligence systems; on the other hand, it has a significant impact on healthcare practices and services at the organisational level, on the actual performance of diagnosis and intervention, and on the rights of individuals, first and foremost the right to health and the right to data protection.

Electronic health records, biomedical imaging, wearable devices, biobanks, medical apps, surgical robots, as well as application of telemedicine and remote monitoring systems are just examples of the elements that are contributing, at a particularly accelerated rate (as demonstrated by the pandemic experience, with the so-called Green Pass), to increase the availability of electronic health data. The arising issue leans on the correct use of health (personal) data for multiple purposes and its protection, which is now increasingly scattered and fragmented among a flood of regulatory measures, which are even more technical and analytical.

One particular aspect to consider is scientific and statistical research, which is essential not only for healthcare but also for science. Research studies can be retrospective or prospective, but in any case, they necessarily require data, personal data, and "sensitive" data (recte "special categories of personal data", as art. 9 GDPR says). In other terms, research today is data centric.

Scientific research is also the primary driver of societal change, with direct repercussions on the whole community and the quality of life of its members, as well as for future generations. The interests underlying scientific activities are balanced with the rights and principles of the individual recognised by the legal system, from both public and private perspectives, which are today recognised also at the constitutional level. The right to data protection, for example, is not an absolute prerogative, but must be considered in light of its social function and balanced with other fundamental rights, in accordance with the principle of proportionality (recital no. 4, GDPR).

Proportionality should often be considered by looking at the means for collecting, processing, and sharing health data that are capable of reconciling individual rights with supra-individual interests. For example, Mission 6 of the Italian National Recovery and Resilience Plan (NRRP), inspired by the principles of "proximity, innovation, and equality", says that health policies should be oriented towards strengthening and enhancing existing infrastructure, such as electronic health records and electronic medical records, which are included in a broader national health data ecosystem. This update—labelled EHR 2.0—is accompanied by the removal of consent regarding the processing of health data: from a "consent-based" vision, in which the individual grants or refuses the transfer of their data, the paradigm shift moves to a more participatory control, in which the individual could intervene directly and immediately in the circulation of their data.

Looking only at the national landscape would certainly be short-sighted. The solution for balancing different fundamental rights and principles can only be achieved through convergent regulation at the supranational level.

As a different model of health data circulation is taking shape, data flow is even more "controlled" rather than "free".

I would like to highlight one of the objectives of the Regulation (EU) 2025/327 of the European Parliament and of the Council of February 11, 2025, on the European Health Data Space, which also aims to enhance cross-border healthcare services, as well as supporting scientific progress in the medical field. The aim is to reduce the scope of regulatory burden and constraints on the (free) flow of data stored in electronic systems. Strengthening the right to portability, consolidating the right of revocation, and reorganising data management systems, based on a functional criterion that reflects the intended use of the data, reflect the idea of a regulated market together with a state intervention.

In this regard, I would like to mention an interesting decision by the Italian Data Protection Authority (no. 465 of September 28, 2023), relating to the PRIMAGE project, with regard to a prior consultation pursuant to Article 110 of the Privacy Code. Here, the legal basis for the transfer of health data in the context of medical, biomedical, and epidemiological research falling within the scope of the EU Horizon project was considered to be the same EU legislation governing the European funding framework programme rather than the consent of the data subject.

Our project fits into this context, which is certainly complex and which I leave to the speakers of the first session to unravel.

The PADS4Health project should be considered for its interdisciplinary path, involving not only law professors but also computer scientists, oncologists, and haematologists. Through a joint action, the goal of the project is to identify a variety of models for facilitating the sharing of health data for scientific research purposes.

Many models could be based on Personal Information Management Systems (PIMS) and Personal Data Store (PDS), well-known—but not widely used—software technologies that allow personal data to be stored in a personal cloud, thus enabling at the same time immediate access to personal data by the data subject and the possibility of selectively granting access to third-party requesters, whether they are medical staff or researchers.

The implications of such models with regard to the GDPR are clear, acting as technical, organisational, and security measures, in compliance with the principles of transparency and security, guaranteeing the practical exercise of individual rights, including those of access, erasure, and portability established by the Regulation. Furthermore, in line with the NRRP objective of seeing the EHR as the single and exclusive point of access for citizens to NHS services, a PDS also seems to be able to easily serve as the main access point for health data sharing.

Let me also say that the most recent EU Regulation refers to these technologies in several places, in accordance with accountability, data protection by design, and so on. This is the case of the Data Governance Act with reference to data intermediaries. Moreover, the EHDS Regulation recognises them as an element that can be linked to the health record and electronic patient record system, to better promote the secondary use of health data. Indeed, it seems clear that a PDS could be the first step towards the creation of a federated data-sharing platform, as well as a concrete application, at least in public administration, of the once-only principle, whereby citizens only provide their data to public authorities once.

Another main issue related to digitalisation in healthcare can be seen in the convergence of various regulatory subsystems, from personal data protection to intellectual property and from contract law to liability law.

It is precisely the latter, which will be explored in depth in the second session, that poses the legal problem of the risk that eHealth technologies could become a means of undermining the therapeutic alliance, which is an immediate corollary of the doctor–patient relationship.

Understanding how the AI system works (the so-called explainability) is far from incapable of influencing and jeopardising not only the health of the individual, but also the operation of the private autonomy and the configurability of the patient's informed consent to medical treatment. Trusting an "opaque" system leads to a new configuration of the doctor–patient relationship, characterised by "machine paternalism" (according to the logic that "computers know best)", which knows everything and decides everything.

In this sense, Article 7, paragraph 3, of the Italian draft law no. 1146-B/2024 on AI states that "the data subject has the right to be informed about the use of artificial intelligence technologies and the advantages, in terms of diagnosis and treatment, deriving from the use of new technologies, as well as to receive information on the decision-making logic used", but paragraph 5 is careful to emphasise that "artificial intelligence systems in healthcare are a support in the processes of prevention, diagnosis, treatment, and therapeutic choice, without prejudice to the final decision, which is always left to medical professionals".

The next steps are to identify the conditions for comprehensible as well as comprehensive information on AI, as well as proportionate, reasonable, and appropriate use of "smart" medical devices, which do not sacrifice certain aspects of our humanity, for medicine "with" machines and not "of" machines.

It is therefore a question not so much of whether to inform or what to inform, but how to inform. In this regard, too, it is clear that technology, and in particular PIMS/PDS, can offer effective support for the protection of individuals.

The awareness—which I would say is still to be fully acquired—is that it is humans who build technology and that it is never a neutral tool.

I would like to thank all the speakers, moderators, and participants and wish you a successful conference.

Venice, Italy Alessandro Bernes

Preface

The project that gave rise to this conference was, first and foremost, a valuable opportunity for us lawyers to engage in dialogue and, above all, to listen to what experts from other fields have to say.

Meetings between legal professionals and experts in the medical and healthcare fields often result in a clash between the former, who invoke the need to safeguard and protect healthcare data, and the latter, who call for greater freedom of action, free from bureaucratic constraints, for purposes that are also in the general interest. Among other things, this conference attempts to provide an initial response to these questions.

We are at an important turning point, in which the European legislator has taken an explicit position on the opportunity and necessity of fully exploiting the potential of data, including in the healthcare field. However, this is not an easy paradigm shift: first of all, the European legislator cannot go back on its word, and, after years of adopting a restrictive position on the processing of personal data, emphasising the risks rather than the benefits, it must be cautious in abandoning the safeguards that have characterised its work to date. Secondly, there is a major problem of trust: after raising awareness of the risks of data processing, citizens need to be reassured that the new direction towards a greater use of data will not be at the expense of their rights and interests, and this is also a delicate operation.

Another area where it is important to build trust is that of artificial intelligence systems. The meeting between lawyers and IT specialists, made possible by this project, is essential in order to make an informed assessment of the adequacy of the regulatory framework established by the European legislator. The use of artificial intelligence systems in the healthcare sector raises delicate issues of liability: these are not new issues, and lawyers are already accustomed to dealing with risk-based liability systems, but it is clear that this requires an understanding of the technical side of the phenomenon. What is new are the kinds of interactions that such systems can have with human beings: here too, it is essential to know how these systems function to understand the actual scope of the anthropocentric principle, which has been repeatedly affirmed by the European legislator.

The following lectures therefore seek to clarify how the transition is taking place, critically outlining its contours in a critical manner. I join Prof. Alessandro Bernes in thanking the colleagues who will participate in this meeting, and I now give the floor to the speakers.

Turin, Italy

Shaira Thobani

About the Book

The book aims to collect the written essays of the keynote speakers who have been part of the event titled "Digitalisation in Health Care Between New Technologies, Data and Research", a conference that was held at Ca' Foscari University of Venice on November 29 and 30, 2024.

The initiative was born as an interdisciplinary workshop, as well as an opportunity for interprofessional dialogue, not only between academics.

The healthcare system has been profoundly revolutionised with the advent of the digital age. In the medical field, however, digitalisation is much more than a technical process: on the one hand, it involves technologies and algorithms, including AI systems; on the other hand, it has a significant impact on health practices and services at an organisational level, on the concrete performance of diagnosis and intervention, and on the rights of natural persons, first and foremost the right to health and the right to data protection.

This study was carried out within the Privacy-Aware Data Sharing model for Health data (PADS4Health) and received funding from the European Union Next-GenerationEU, National Recovery and Resilience Plan (NRRP), Mission 4, Component 2, and Investiment 1.1 Fondo per il Programma Nazionale di Ricerca e Progetti di Rilevante Interesse Nazionale (PRIN), CUP N. H53D23010880001. This manuscript reflects only the authors' views and opinions; neither the European Union nor the European Commission can be considered responsible for them.

Contents

Editors and Contributors

About the Editors

Alessandro Bernes, Ph.D., is an assistant professor of Private Law at the Department of Economics, Ca' Foscari University of Venice. He has substantial experience in legal issues related to data processing for scientific, historical, and statistical research purposes. His studies focus on how to foster research data sharing by implementing technical and organisational measures in order to better ensure the protection of individuals. He has published articles and essays in various scientific academic journals on personal data protection, and he has also co-authored a book on privacy and data protection in software services for an international publisher. He is the principal investigator of the Italian project of national interest PRIN 2022 PNRR "PADS4Health".

Shaira Thobani, Ph.D., is an associate professor at the Department of Law, University of Turin. She has extensive experience with data protection and management issues addressed from a private law perspective. In this field, her main research areas include the requirements for consent of the data subject to be valid, the market of personal data, and the private law remedies (civil liability) in case of violation of the right to personal data protection. She is also an associate principal investigator of the Italian project of national interest PRIN 2022 PNRR "PADS4Health".

Contributors

Luca Bolognini Lawyer, Italian Institute for Privacy and Data Valorisation, Milan, Italy

Valentina Calderai Associate Professor of Comparative Private Law, University of Pisa, Pisa, Italy

Stefano Campostrini Full Professor of Social Statistics, Ca' Foscari University of Venice, Venice, Italy

Martina D'Onofrio Assistant Professor of Private Law, University of Milano-Bicocca, Milan, Italy

Roberto D'Orazio Permanent Official, Office for Foreign Legislation of the Chamber of Deputies, Rome, Italy

Mirko Faccioli Associate Professor of Private Law, University of Verona, Verona, Italy

Massimo Foglia Associate Professor of Private Law, University of Bergamo, Bergamo, Italy

Carlotta De Menech Associate Professor of Private Law, University of Pavia, Pavia, Italy

Salvatore Orlando Full Professor of Private Law, Sapienza University of Rome, Rome, Italy

Beniamino Parenzo Research Grant Holder, Ca' Foscari University of Venice, Venice, Italy

Alessandra Poggiani Director General, Consorzio CINECA, Bologna, Italy

Vincenzo Ricciuto Full Professor of Private Law, Tor Vergata University of Rome, Rome, Italy

Giovanni Di Rosa Full Professor of Private Law, University of Catania, Catania, Italy

Chiara Di Somma Officer, Office of the Italian Data Protection Authority, Rome, Italy

Francesco Giacomo Viterbo Full Professor of Private Law, University of Salento, Lecce, Italy

Part I
Digital Healthcare, Personal Data Processing and Scientific Research

Chapter 1
Health Data Regulation: Normative Innovations and Comparative Perspectives

Roberto D'Orazio

1 The Digitalisation of Health Data

The regulation of health data has long, and increasingly, engaged the attention of constitutional and comparative law scholars, guiding their reflections along two principal lines of inquiry. On the one hand, their focus has turned to the innovative aspects—and the related challenges—that the digitalisation of such data entails for the promotion and protection of fundamental rights. On the other hand, they have considered the consequences that the digitalisation process may produce, particularly in States with a regional or federal structure, in terms of the distribution of legislative competences. From this perspective, scholars have asked whether, and to what extent, the digital transition might result in a formal or substantive centralisation of powers in the hands of the central state authorities (or even of the European Union), relegating local governments to the mere implementation of rules defined elsewhere; or whether, by contrast, effective coordination between different levels of government may instead be a viable and preferable objective.

These macro-profiles trace the general coordinates of "digital health", understood as the reference framework of the institutional and regulatory arrangement that is gradually taking shape with regard to the protection and circulation of personal health data. The degree of complexity of this framework is determined precisely by aspects relating to the protection of fundamental rights and by the convergence of legal texts, articulated on the grounds of multilevel sources and of internal distribution of competences within States.

R. D'Orazio (✉)
Office for Foreign Legislation of the Chamber of Deputies, Rome, Italy

A. Bernes, S. Thobani (eds.), *Digitalisation in Health Care between New Technologies, Data and Research*, Services and Business Process Reengineering, https://doi.org/10.1007/978-981-95-6982-3_1

A general metaphor that has gained widespread acceptance in describing the legal space in which personal data are situated and circulate is that of the ecosystem, a notion now entered into general use. Borrowed from the natural sciences, this term designates an environment shaped by the interactions taking place within it, whose overall balance results from the relationships established among its various components. One may likewise speak of the existence of a health data ecosystem, endowed with specific characteristics by virtue of the interests involved and on account of the overlap of regulatory competences. This ecosystem is governed by a dual set of rules: those applicable to the special categories of data (Art. 9 GDPR), which include health data, and those which, within the welfare state, shape the organisation required to ensure the effectiveness of the right to health—a right whose fundamental character is significantly indicated by the fact that, in the Italian Constitution, it is the only right expressly qualified as such (Art. 32).

The defining features of the health data ecosystem (a notion now codified in EU legislation) can be inferred from the legal indicators that both delineate its boundaries and evolve in response to its developmental stage, propelled by the digital transition. This latter term, while commonly used, assumes a specific connotation in the legal context. Here, "transition" does not merely denote a general openness to change—regarded as inherent to the law—but refers to the urgent need for legislation to anticipate and channel certain societal transformations, intervening ex ante to guide and shape their trajectories. This is precisely the meaning of the "digital transition" pursued in the health sector by European Union legislation, whose overarching objective is to enhance citizens' health by improving the efficiency of healthcare systems.

Personal data represent the unifying element of this evolutionary path of European law; indeed, it may be said that, within this context, they perform a genuinely regulatory function. This function is rooted in the Charter of Fundamental Rights of the European Union, where data protection (Art. 8) is established as the foundation of a normative triangle, whose other vertices are the dignity of the individual (Art. 1) and the freedom to conduct a business (Art. 16).

The defined legal status of personal data and their centrality in the digital health framework make them a key reference point for any coherent interpretation of this field of law—especially when contrasted with the blurred boundaries that still characterise the notions of "digitalisation" and "digital transformation". Nothwistanding that these concepts are recurrent in the formulation of both European and national public policies, they still lack a stable and universally accepted definition. Indeed, it seems clear that such definitions, although closely connected to the operation of digital infrastructures, cannot be reduced to their technological foundations alone. Rather, they must be framed within the context of State activities and considered in light of constitutional and administrative rules aimed at innovating, developing and managing the operation and performance of public administrations—whether in their internal procedures, in the delivery of public services, or in their interaction with citizens and businesses.

2 The European Health Data Space

Within this general framework, the digitalisation of health data—which not only constitutes a form of processing in itself but typically paves the way for further uses—has sparked a cascade of regulatory innovations.

It should be noted that the issue of secondary use of data has emerged, from the outset, as a matter of critical importance for the very effectiveness of data protection rules. Such processing occupies a somewhat eccentric position within the architecture of the protection system, whose keystone is the principle of purpose limitation. According to this principle, and subject to narrowly defined exceptions, it is generally inadmissible the use personal data for purposes other than those that justified their initial collection and for which consent—where required—was obtained.

Nonetheless, the GDPR provides for certain derogations and relaxations of this principle in the context of scientific research, in recognition of its methodological specificities, inherent need for personal data, and overarching social value. Moreover, the normative caution traditionally shown toward the secondary use of data has had to confront increasing pressure from the most innovation-driven sectors of the economy and research—particularly those aligned with the European Union's policy agenda for the digitalisation of health data.

Such is the rationale underlying Regulation 2025/327, which establishes the *European Health Data Space* (EHDS): a set of legal provisions, norms, and common practices, converging in establishing an overall governance for both the primary and secondary use of personal electronic health data. This category of data, characterised by the close link to the individual's private sphere, as well as by the digital format and standardised criteria for their processing, storage, and circulation, constitutes a particular variant (though one likely to become predominant over time) of the broader category of "data concerning health" included among the "special categories of data" under Art. 9 of the GDPR.

One of the innovative aspects of the EHDS Regulation lies in the way it specifies and contextualises the general principles governing the processing and circulation of personal data, in order to transpose them into a sector characterised by the interplay of multiple "sensitive" interests and by the complexity of the necessary balancing operations. The result is a detailed regulatory setting in which the individual's interest in retaining control over their personal data intersects with the interest in sharing such data to promote medical and scientific research and improve healthcare methods and their management. Within this framework, the fundamental right to health coexists with the development of the healthcare services market—an interaction also reflected in the dual legal basis of the founding regulation, grounded in Art. 16 and 114 of the TFEU.

The emerging system built around the EHDS thus identifies the processing of health data as a pivotal instrument through which, under appropriate safeguards, both scientific research and access to healthcare services for citizens can be facilitated and enhanced. This regulatory process, however, forms part of a broader strategy. Its guiding framework is the European Union's digital transformation agenda launched over the past 5 years, which, it is worth recalling, envisions the adoption of no fewer than 23 legislative acts by 2030 (some already adopted, others still under negotiation or in draft form), all converging toward the goal of promoting and realising the development and competitiveness of "common European sectoral spaces".

This ambitious legislative plan already includes regulatory measures aimed at building a data-driven economy, as outlined in the *Data Governance Act* (Regulation 2022/868) and the forthcoming *Data Act*—two horizontal instruments that establish general rules applicable also to the health sector. These must be added to the *Interoperable Europe Act* (Regulation 2023/2854), which enables national administrations to cooperate in delivering public services across territorial, sectoral, and organisational borders, while preserving sovereignty at each level of governance. Neither can the *AI Act* (Regulation 2024/1689) be overlooked. As is well known, its provisions regulate the use of artificial intelligence systems through a horizontal, technology-neutral approach, based on risk assessment; therefore, this framework helps shape the regulatory environment in which AI systems are deployed in healthcare and biomedical contexts. Particular attention must also be given to the normative instruments addressing data security. These include Directive 2022/2555 on the security of network and information systems (NIS2), the *Cyber Resilience Act* (Regulation 2024/2847), and the *Cyber Solidarity Act* (Regulation 2025/38). The former strengthens cybersecurity standards for products incorporating digital components, imposing security-by-design obligations on manufacturers. The latter, by contrast, focuses on large-scale cyberattacks and emergency response mechanisms, complementing the preventive approach of the former.

The overarching goal of this extensive legislative activity—which underscores the strategic value now attributed to data (including non-personal data) and to the infrastructures necessary for their circulation—is to define a coherent regulatory context for the efficient management and sharing of data within the public sector and between public and private actors. This goal cannot disregard the implications for fundamental rights—given that the success of the European model as a global normative reference depends on striking an effective balance between technological innovation and the protection of rights in the healthcare domain.

3 The Protection of Fundamental Rights

Here, then, is the first key point. From the perspective of the protection of fundamental rights, the digitalisation of health data presents itself as a dual-faced phenomenon. On the one hand, it amplifies the risks to which personal data are exposed. Their legal protection is challenged by digitalisation procedures, which, behind an ostensibly unified label, in fact consist of multiple phases and segments. In relation to each of these, verifying the compliance of individual processing operations with data protection rules can at times prove difficult—yet such verification is all the more necessary when, due to certain purposes and conditions of processing, the general framework allows for the application of exceptions and derogations.

The other side of the coin lies not in the potential vulnerability of the individuals arising from the digitalisation of their health data, but in the significant advantages that it may bring for the exercise of their right to health.

A paradigmatic example is offered by the use—following initial experimentation in industrial sectors—of the so-called *Digital Twin* (or *Virtual Human Twin*) model in the biomedical field. These are virtual representations of a person capable of reproducing their anatomical, pathophysiological, and cognitive features, thus enabling the monitoring of vital functions and health status, the development of personalised pharmacological treatments, and the planning and simulation of surgical interventions to be later carried out in vivo. The "twinning" process is made possible by the continuous flow of data from the physical individual to their digital counterpart, supported by technologies such as the Internet of Things (IoT), Artificial Intelligence (AI), machine learning, and imaging techniques. These allow for ongoing interaction, communication, and synchronisation between the individual and their digital twin, such that the latter constantly and dynamically reflects the condition of the real person. As a result, healthcare professionals are able to rely on rapid and reliable decision-making processes.

This is a technology whose complexity has not escaped the attention of legal scholars, who have identified issues that extend beyond data protection to include questions of ownership. They have in fact asked whether the person subjected to the twinning system might claim respect for their digital identity and claim exclusive rights over the digital prototype; and even without delving here into the proprietary or contractual implications of the matter, it is evident that these issues are of legal relevance—unless one were to assume that the individual concerned has no say in the fate of their digital twin, like Peter Schlemihl deprived of his shadow in the famous tale by von Chamisso.

What is important to note at this stage is that the creation and operation of these systems presuppose the existence and accessibility of vast repositories of health data—derived, for instance, from electronic health records or obtained from patients' genetic, physical, and biological characteristics. It is therefore evident that the development of such promising technology requires an advanced regulatory framework, one capable of facilitating—while safeguarding individual rights—the integration of diverse datasets for the sharing of high-quality and sufficiently heterogeneous data. Such integration is essential during the model training phase to ensure that the broadest possible range of cases is taken into account.

From this perspective, the requirements imposed by the GDPR for the processing of health-related data—stricter than those for ordinary data—may act as a constraint on the development of these new systems, even when such development is to be supported through so-called data altruism (now envisaged by the EHDS Regulation as operating by default, unless the individual opts out), and has to be pursued in the name of the solidarity principle where expressly enshrined in constitutional charters.

Moreover, while the European legislator has established uniform and directly applicable data protection rules across all Member States, it has also left room for national lawmakers to adapt these rules within their domestic legal systems, including, with respect to provisions on special categories of data such as health data. As a result, divergent interpretations and implementations of the GDPR have led to a fragmentation and differentiation of national legal frameworks, which negatively impact the effective interoperability and standardisation of such data.

This is a crucial aspect. If the European legislator has aimed to enhance the value of data by promoting its circulation and sharing, then standardisation and interoperability represent the necessary technological complements to this effort. It is also essential—as recently emphasised in the Draghi Report on EU Competitiveness (2024)—to consider the risks posed by regulatory fragmentation, which may create or exacerbate disparities among Member States. It is not accidental that even a brief comparative overview of the legal frameworks and organisational models adopted in some Member States may reveal that some countries, by making more effective use of health data for planning and managing healthcare services, are better equipped than others to meet citizens' expectations and to do so in a more financially sustainable manner.

These challenges help to explain developments that have occurred both in practice and in regulation. At the level of operational rules, the use of synthetic data has gained traction, supported also by European initiatives. Synthetic data refers to data artificially generated through the use of advanced algorithms and machine learning techniques to create datasets that replicate the characteristics of real data without revealing sensitive or personal information. The aim is to preserve the statistical integrity and analytical utility of the original data while avoiding the constraints associated with the use of personal or otherwise identifiable data. When properly generated, synthetic data shares the essential properties of anonymous data, as it is not linked to any individual and does not lend itself to re-identification processes. Evidence of this equivalence can be found in the AI Act, which, under Art. 10, lists the circumstances in which the use of sensitive personal data (such as health data) is permitted for bias detection. It explicitly requires that such use be allowed only where the detection and correction of bias cannot be effectively achieved using other data, including synthetic or anonymised data. Similarly, Art. 59 of the same legislative act provides that the processing of personal data within a regulatory sandbox is permissible only when the use of "synthetic, anonymous, or other non-personal data" would not fulfil the same objectives.

From a regulatory standpoint, the aforementioned EHDS Regulation therefore is the cornerstone of the European data strategy and stands out as the first legislative instrument aimed at establishing a common data space in a specific sector. Leaving aside a detailed examination of its provisions, it is worth noting that its core focus lies in the regulation of both the primary and secondary use of health data. The primary use refers to the provision of healthcare services to the individual to whom the data pertain; the secondary use is aimed, in essence, at resolving the uncertainties cast by the GDPR over such further use of personal data, particularly given the principle of purpose limitation and the limited recognition it gives to "further processing".

This regulatory approach reflects the dual objective underlying the rules on the protection and circulation of health data: on the one hand, to safeguard a fundamental right of the individual; on the other hand, to enable the sharing and portability of such data, albeit under the individual's control. What is thereby established is a dialectical relationship not only between the individual and the market, but also between the protection of individual rights and the pursuit of the public interest. In other words, the valorization of data in the health and biomedical domain is relevant not only—or not primarily—from an economic standpoint, as it also matters in respect to the fulfilment of the public interest. This latter aspect, it must be recalled, is a condition for the lawfulness of data processing for secondary purposes and is closely tied to the "social function" of the right to personal data protection, as affirmed by the GDPR.

3.1 National Legislative Developments

The trend described above can also be observed in domestic legal developments, which reflect a repositioning of the public interest in relation to the processing of health data. In this regard, the Italian legal framework may serve as a reference point. It has recently been revised through an amendment to the Personal Data Protection Code (the "Codice in materia di protezione dei dati personali"), aimed at facilitating the processing of data for scientific research purposes. Under the new regime, such processing may now take place without the need for prior consultation with the national supervisory authority (Art. 110); the authority instead plays a role in defining up-to-date ethical guidelines for processing activities conducted for scientific research purposes. To further simplify the legal landscape, another legislative amendment (to Art. 2-*sexies* of the aforementioned Code) has introduced the general administrative act, alongside statutory law, as a valid legal basis for processing activities carried out in the execution of a task in the public interest—including the processing of special categories of data for public health purposes.

In the same direction—strengthening the recognition of the public interest in the circulation and sharing of health data—moves the Law on Artificial Intelligence (n. 132/2005) approved by the Italian Parliament on September 2025, conferring the Government delegate powers to issue legislative decrees in the field of AI systems (and thus to adopt provisions whose full compatibility with the self-executing provisions of the AI Act may need to be verified, in the opinion of some scholars). This Law expressly recognises the "significant public interest" of the processing of data - including special categories of data - carried out by public bodies and by non-profit private entities for purposes of scientific research and experimentation aimed at developing artificial intelligence systems for healthcare and biomedical use. In this way, the Law establishes and clarifies the legal basis for such processing, grounded on the constitutional principles affirming the fundamental right to health as well as the freedom of research and culture (Art. 32 and 33, Italian constitution).

Within the current legislative agenda, some other initiatives also deserve attention, at least as indicators of the current perception of the state of "digital healthcare" and its future prospects. In Italy, some bills (under parliamentary consideration at the time of writing) aim to amend the rules governing health data in order to promote scientific research and, consequently, to achieve results that may enhance the protection of citizens' health. These proposals envisage the introduction of experimental research activities based on health data to be conducted in a secure environment modelled on the concept of a regulatory sandbox. Such an environment would allow for the protection of patients' privacy while also helping to overcome the rigidities of GDPR application.

Regardless of their specific content, these initiatives are valuable insofar as they highlight the need for regulatory tools suited to testing preventive and therapeutic solutions that can be applied in situations—such as emergencies or epidemics—typically requiring rapid intervention, which traditional authorisation procedures for the use of health data for research and public health may not allow.

4 Multilevel Normative Frameworks

The second aspect to be considered concerns the existence of multiple regulatory sources and the effects that the distribution of normative competences produces in the context of health data digitalisation. This is a matter of undeniable significance in States whose institutional organisation is based on the allocation of powers between central government and territorial autonomies. The impact of digitalisation on subnational levels of government can be assessed, from different analytical standpoints, either as a factor likely to diminish the pluralism inherent in systems of territorial self-government, or as a potential obstacle to the adoption of uniform procedural standards on which the efficiency of public administrations depends.

Once again, digitalisation reveals its twofold nature. The standardisation of rules and processes may constrain institutional diversity in ways more subtle than explicit centralisation, and may unfold independently of formal relations between levels of government or undelying power-allocation dynamics. Where it is not the central State restricting the competences of territorial entities, nor the European Union extending its remit at the expense of Member States, it is the private sector that stands to gain from a transfer of authority from public institutions. Private actors, in fact, are capable of achieving this result through the definition of digital standards that become applicable across the public sphere, irrespective of the level of government involved. This development raises serious concerns about the effectiveness of public oversight over private power and the State's capacity to shape the digital domain, an increasingly central arena for the exercise of governmental functions and for virtually all forms of social activity.

In relation to these issues, valuable insights may be drawn from the examination of some national experiences. Although commonly reported as a successful case of digital transition in the public sector, the Estonian example proves to be of limited usefulness for the purposes of this analysis. In that context, the extensive digitalisation of public life has been facilitated by a high degree of social homogeneity and by the emphasis placed on national identity—an emphasis that is understandable in light of the country's historical and political background. Of greater relevance are the experiences of Italy and Germany, both of which have recently witnessed a tendency toward the vertical consolidation of regulatory competences, brought about, respectively, by the implementation of the "National Recovery and Resilience Plan" (*Piano Nazionale di Ripresa e Resilienza*, PNRR) and by legislation concerning the digitalisation of public administration.

In neither case is there an explicit constitutional attribution of legislative competence regarding the digitalisation of public administration. The issue is not specifically addressed at the constitutional level, except for the protection of citizens' data and their right to information expressly provided by the *Grundesetz*. However, Germany amended the *Grundgesetz* in 2017 by introducing a provision granting the Federation (*Bund*) the competence to regulate "comprehensive electronic access to the administrative services of the federal and *Länder* governments by means of a federal law with the consent of the *Bundesrat*" (Art. 91c, para. 5). As part of the implementation of this constitutional reform, the Online Access Act (*Onlinezugangsgesetz*—OZG) was adopted the same year, aiming to establish a framework for cooperation among public administrations. To this end, the Act requires both the Federation and the *Länder* to provide their services also in digital format and to ensure the interoperability of their information systems.

The Italian case seems also significant from the perspective of the relationship between composite statehood and healthcare universalism. The pandemic brought to light the critical issues arising from the organisational autonomy of the regions in the field of healthcare. Regional autonomy does not appear to have sufficiently ensured — neither in the pre-pandemic phase, nor during the emergency, nor even in the aftermath—the development of uniform technological tools enabling effective interoperability and cooperation among healthcare services in different regions - and, at times, even within the same region.

It is therefore unsurprising that healthcare digitalisation is increasingly seen as the principal path toward greater efficiency and cost-effectiveness in the delivery of healthcare services. Moreover, the adoption of new technologies in the health sector is now also incentivised by the objectives outlined in the aforementioned PNRR, which repeatedly emphasises the centrality of digitalization particularly within "Mission 6", which states that "the plan decisively accelerates the improvement, harmonisation, and dissemination of the Electronic Health Record as a cornerstone for the provision of digital health services and the valorisation of national clinical data".

Further complicating the overall framework are the current proposals for constitutional reform aimed at recognising differentiated regional autonomy (in implementation of Art. 116, para. 3, of the Italian Constitution). It is the subject of ongoing debate whether the recognition of such autonomy could help bridge the existing gap between regions in the provision of healthcare services. Consistent with expectations, this gap has been a central point of criticism in public discourse among those opposed to "differentiated regionalism" (namely, the attribution of a higher level of autonomy to regions that meet specific criteria); they argue that this may risk increasing inequalities in access to healthcare across the country. Supporters of the reform, on the other hand, counter that maintaining the current system would result in a levelling-down of healthcare provision across the national territory, ultimately stifling the excellence and innovation achieved by certain local and regional health systems.

However, the unifying role of technological infrastructure—particularly in the field of public healthcare—does not appear to have received due attention in current debates on the matter. Yet it is precisely in this domain that technology could give concrete expression to the constitutional principles of unity and indivisibility of the Republic (as enshrined in Art. 5 of the Italian Constitution). This prospect, in my view, can be grounded in Art. 117, para. 2, (r) of the Italian Constitution, which does not explicitly refer to digitalisation—neither in its broader sense, nor specifically in relation to the organisation of public administration. Nevertheless, it entrusts the State with exclusive legislative competence over all technological aspects, insofar as it refers to the "statistical and IT coordination of data of state, regional and local administrations". Admittedly, this wording may be considered insufficient to clearly encompass within the scope of "statistical and IT coordination of data" the modern concepts of "digitalisation" or "digital transition". On the other hand, the State's coordinating role in this domain could, in principle, be reconciled with a residual legislative competence of the Regions for all aspects falling outside the scope of such coordination. It should also be noted that the Constitutional Court has so far adopted a restrictive interpretation of this area of State competence, limiting it to strictly technical interventions aimed at "ensuring a commonality of language, procedures, and uniform standards, so as to enable interoperability among the information systems of the public administration" (Judgment No. 17/2004).

Nevertheless, the most recent developments in the field seem to point towards its reclassification as an area falling under the full legislative competence of the central State, also in light of the growing influence of European Union law. Indeed, it is necessary to take into account the substantial evolution in the scope of the subject matters listed in Art. 117 of the Constitution, a development that also reflects broader societal changes. Digital transition is perhaps the area in which this phenomenon is most evident, by virtue of its systemic nature—insofar as it brings about a socio-cultural transition capable of reshaping the role of the physician, the doctor–patient relationship, and even the very concepts of medicine and health. It therefore appears reasonable to assume that the aforementioned subject matter—falling within the scope of "State coordination" and understood in its broadest sense—has undergone a process of progressive expansion in both reach and impact. This may be sufficient to argue for assigning to the State the competence to govern the "digital transition", or at the very least, to qualify it as a "transversal" matter—particularly where it intersects with the protection of health, an area of concurrent competence between the State and the Regions.

From a preliminary examination of some of the most significant national models (to which one might add the case of Austria, where the federal structure of the State is accompanied by a tendency to centralise relevant legislative competences on digitalisation in the hands of the *Bund*, pursuant to federal administrative procedure law), it emerges that in systems where legislative responsibility is in some way shared between a state and sub-state level, there is a consistent need to ensure coordination through the higher level of government. However, this often results in a potential tendency toward excessive centralisation, either through amendments to the constitutional legal framework, as exemplified by the German case, or through the expansion of central government powers via judicial interpretation, as in the Italian case.

5 Concluding Remarks

The reflections presented above highlight the complexity and strategic significance of the legal framework governing the use of health data. While the protection of personal data remains a fundamental value within the European legal order, the emerging regulatory trend—both at the EU and national levels—reveals a growing awareness of the need to reconcile this protection with the promotion of innovation, scientific research, and the public interest.

The initiatives undertaken at the European level, notably through the GDPR, the AI Act, and the EHDS Regulation, as well as those being developed within national legislations, signal a progressive shift towards enabling data access and reuse under conditions of trust, transparency, and accountability. Central to this evolving framework is the recognition that high-quality, interoperable, and representative datasets are indispensable for the training of trustworthy AI systems, and that legal certainty is essential for their responsible development and deployment.

In this context, the use of synthetic data, regulatory sandboxes, and the explicit identification of public interest as a legal basis for processing special categories of data represent promising tools for bridging the gap between data protection and data-driven innovation. However, such tools must be carefully calibrated to ensure that the fundamental rights of individuals are not compromised, and that the collective benefits of data use are fairly distributed across Member States and social groups.

Ultimately, the challenge for lawmakers and regulators lies in designing a legal ecosystem that is not only compliant and secure, but also agile, forward-looking, and capable of supporting the transformative potential of digital health technologies, particularly in view of future public health crises and the increasing demand for personalised and efficient care.

Moreover, the metaphor of the ecosystem—now elevated to a normative concept—recalls the imperative of its overall sustainability. This, too, is a notion of our time. Applied across a wide range of contexts, it shares a common denominator in the responsible use of resources—in this case, personal health data—in ways that preserve essential balances, the disruption of which could destabilise the system as a whole. In European law, such equilibrium finds its guiding star in the principle of human dignity.

Clearly, the path to balance lies along a narrow ridge: on one side are the benefits to be gained from advancing tools for care and research; and on the other side, the risk of undermining personal self-determination—particularly where individuals may find themselves engaged in care relationships shaped by the opaque responses of inscrutable black boxes, without a framework of effective safeguards. Among these, the first and most indispensable is the centrality of the human element.

Bibliography

1. Bolognini L, Zipponi S (eds) (2024) Privacy e diritto dei dati sanitari. Giuffrè Francis Lefebvre, Milano
2. Ciancimino M (2020) Protezione e controllo dei dati in ambito sanitario e intelligenza artificiale. Edizioni Scientifiche Italiane, Napoli
3. De Ruijter A (2019) EU health & policy. The expansion of EU power in public health and health care. Oxford University Press, Oxford
4. Happacher E, Zwilling C, Bußjäger P, Obwexer W, Parolari S (eds) (2025) Digitalisierung und regionale Autonomie. Nomos, Baden-Baden
5. Mărcuţ M (2020) The governance of digital policies. Towards a new competence in the European Union. Palgrave Macmillan, London
6. Sarra C, Zilio A, De Bona G (2025) Diritto alla salute, protezione dei dati e intelligenza artificiale. FrancoAngeli, Milano
7. Thiene A, Corso S (eds) (2023) Protezione dei dati sanitari. Privacy e innovazione tecnologica salute pubblica e diritto alla riservatezza. Jovene, Napoli

Chapter 2
The Legal Basis of Health Data Regulation in the European Sharing Area

Vincenzo Ricciuto

1 Foreword: The Dual Legal Basis in the EHDS

The topic of the "legal basis" of the processing of health data requires us to dwell on how the "legal bases" are understood in the "Regulation (EU) 2025/327 of the European Parliament and of the Council of 11 February 2025 on the European Health Data Space and amending Directive 2011/24/EU and Regulation (EU) 2024/2847" (so-called EHDS).

This is the first common European data space in a specific sector and is part of the European data strategy, representing another step in defining the digital market framework. This space, which constitutes one of the priorities of the European Commission in the health sector, will be an integral part of the construction of a European Health Union. It aims to guarantee access by every individual to their data in electronic format, enable easy sharing with health professionals, and ensure control over their own data, within a framework of interoperability and security.

The phenomenon, then, noting that information and communication technologies have also revolutionised the world of healthcare, can therefore be observed and described—for the purposes that interest us most—in a twofold and competing direction.

V. Ricciuto (✉)
Tor Vergata University of Rome, Rome, Italy
e-mail: vincenzo.ricciuto@uniroma2.it

A. Bernes, S. Thobani (eds.), *Digitalisation in Health Care between New Technologies, Data and Research*, Services and Business Process Reengineering, https://doi.org/10.1007/978-981-95-6982-3_2

2 The Legal Basis Offered by Artt. 16 and 114 TFEU

The first way in which one can speak of "legal basis" concerns the rules (of the Treaties) that legitimise the regulatory intervention of the European institutions.

From the civil law perspective, therefore, it is necessary, first of all, to ask "why" and "how" the discipline in question was introduced by the Regulation, given that the European legislator does not have direct jurisdiction in matters of health, health policies, or health services, which must instead be regulated by individual national laws.

In this regard, as is well known, Artt. 16 and 114 of the TFEU come to the fore. These are rules that, recurring constantly in all the European Regulations on the subject of data (from the GDPR to the AI Act), serve, on the one hand, to ensure the protection of personal data and, on the other, to introduce—and this is one of the fundamental points—the market theme.

A dual legal basis is possible insofar as the regulatory intervention simultaneously pursues multiple objectives that are inextricably linked, with none being secondary or only indirectly connected to the others.

Indeed, Art. 114 TFEU aims to improve the functioning of the internal market through measures for the approximation of national rules; it provides the essential legal foundation enabling the European legislator to intervene in areas where it would otherwhise lack legitimacy. This provision, moreover, stipulates, corsivo, that in achieving harmonisation of the laws, regulations, and administrative provisions of the Member States in the fields of health, safety, environmental protection, and consumer protection, "a high level of protection shall be ensured, taking account, in particular, of any new developments based on scientific facts".

This principle also reflects what is laid down in Art. 168 TFEU, which provides that, in defining and implementing all policies activities of the Union, a "high level of protection of human health is ensured" and that Union action respects "the responsibilities of the Member States for the definition of their health policy and for the organisation and delivery of health services and medical care". Here, the internal market perspective ("European health data space") emerges clearly and explicitly, as health products and services based on data are often developed using electronic health data from different Member States and subsequently marketed throughout the EU.

Historically, the debate surrounding personal data focused, inter alia and beyond the strictly personalistic dimension (namely, the protection of the economic value of an "asset," now central to modern economies), on their circulation and negotiability.

In the same perspective, within EHDS, the issue of electronic health records emerges—as will be seen below—allowing the European legislator to regulate and standardise the rules of the system (making them directly applicable in the individual Member States) with a view to the market, the protection of competition and the circulation of these specific categories of asset.

This justifies and legitimises European regulatory intervention in national legal systems, which, in the absence of a market perspective, would have had exclusive competence in healthcare matters.

As for the second legal basis Art. 16 TFEU comes into play, which states that "everyone has the right to the protection of personal data concerning him or her". Electronic health data, of course, are "sensitive" or, in the GDPR's sense, "special" categories of personal data, so the aspects of the Regulation concerning their processing fall within the scope of EU data protection legislation.

And, however, Art. 9 GDPR in principle restricts the processing of such data, allowing it, for example, on the basis of the explicit consent of the data subject or under other conditions outlined therein, some of which are clearly relevant in the health sector (consider, for instance, the cases referred to in Art. 9(1)(c)(h)(i) GDPR).

The new Health Data Regulation, then, aims to expand the use and processing of those particular data that constitute by electronic health data.

This profile thus makes it possible to address the other way of understanding the "legal basis" within the Regulation.

3 The Legal Basis for the Processing of Health Data

The second way—in addition to the previous one—of referring to a "legal basis" concerns the elements that make the processing of health data lawful, given that the principle of the "dissemination" of electronic health data is emerging, as stated in Recital no. 36 of the EHDS. Indeed, "in order to enable the continuous exchange of electronic health data and to ensure that the rights of individuals and health professionals are respected, electronic health record systems marketed in the internal market should be capable of storing and transmitting, in a secure manner, high quality electronic health data". Furthermore, it is specified that "it is an essential objective of the European Health Data Area to ensure the free and secure flow of electronic health data within the Union".

In this regard, the Regulation distinguishes between a primary and a secondary use of electronic health data.

The "primary use" refers to "the processing of electronic health data for the provision of healthcare in order to assess, maintain or restore the state of health of the natural person to whom such data relate, including the prescription, dispensing and supply of medicines and medical devices, as well as for relevant social, administrative or reimbursement services" (Art. 2(d)).

Therefore, in this case, the issue of the "uploading" (which, as is evident, is a form of "processing") of electronic health data on the platform comes to the fore, but with respect to this processing (which may give rise, if necessary, to the liability of the healthcare facility in the event of erroneous or incomplete uploading of the health data of the person concerned), a problem of "consent" of the person concerned does not arise—as will be immediately stated—according to the traditional logic with which the civil law expert are familiar.

The Regulation, on this point, merely governs the rights of individuals in relation to the primary use of their electronic personal health data, such as (by way of example) the right to access their electronic personal health data, to download an electronic copy free of charge, to grant access to all or part of their electronic personal health data to another healthcare provider of their choice, to restrict healthcare professionals' and healthcare providers' access to all or part of their electronic personal health data, and to obtain information on access to the data by healthcare providers and professionals (Art. 3 ff.).

In this context, the issue also involves the further dissemination of health data to other subjects, since the Regulation governs the direct access by health professionals to personal electronic health data (Art. 11), so that it could be said that the Regulation would seem to authorise corsivo access such data by professionals.

In the present case no form of consent on the part of the data subject is at issue: the Regulation does not require it; and in fact "the legislation of the Member States may [only] provide that natural persons have the right to exclude access to their personal electronic health data recorded in an electronic health record system through electronic health record access services" (Art. 10).

Therefore, it would appear that we are witnessing the transition from a system (typical of the GDPR) where the (subjective) right to processing and the consent of the individual assumed a central and preponderant value, to one in which the "relationship" between the data subject and the data controller is constructed in terms of the former's "burden" to exclude others from the processing of his electronic health data.

It follows that, from the perspective of market protection, the rule that is asserting itself with increasing force is that of the circulation, access and sharing of this particular category of data, with the burden placed on the data subject to express dissent; dissent that is tantamount to excluding from processing all subjects other than those who are obliged to upload electronic health data.

Upstream reflection cannot then disregard either the issue of the value of consent (its manifestation in a free, specific, informed, and unequivocal form) particularly within the context of new technologies.

As anticipated, the truth is that the regulation on the primary use of health data aims to ensure the circulation at European level, also thanks to the experience of the "electronic health record". These electronic health records document the destination and use of relevant health data, achieving the 'single market of health data' regardless of the consent (traditionally understood) of the data subject to the processing of personal data.

As to the "secondary use" emerges, instead, "the processing of electronic health data for the purposes indicated in Chapter IV of … the regulation, which are different from the initial purposes for which such data were collected or produced" (Art. 2(e)).

In particular (Art. 53), this includes processing for purposes of public interest in the field of public health or occupational medicine; policy-making and regulatory activities in support of public bodies or Union institutions, bodies, and organs;

statistics; education or teaching activities in the health sector; scientific research in the health or welfare sector.

With regard to the secondary use of electronic health data, a fundamental role is played by the institution of data authorisation, which, according to Art. 68, is issued by the body responsible, upon application and following the assessment of a number of requirements.

Ultimately, the regulation creates a European health data space in which individuals can easily control their electronic health data.

A "space", an internal market for health data, emerges through express legal provision. These data are subject to processing which, for certain hypotheses, finds its "legal basis" in a "legal obligation"; for others, in the performance of public interest tasks (as is the case for the MyHealth@EU infrastructure: "this regulation", states Recital 34, "constitutes the legal basis for the processing of electronic personal health data in MyHealth@EU (MyHealth@EU) as a task carried out in the public interest assigned by Union law pursuant to Art. 6(1)(e) of Regulation (EU) 2016/679"; and, regarding healthcare provided using personal data, in the "necessity" of carrying out the processing for medical purposes (Art. 9(h) GDPR).

The data subject, consequently, will only be able to oppose, if and when the relevant discipline aimed at concretely allowing the exercise of the "right of exclusion" is adopted in the individual Member States.

The topic, again, intercepts the relationship between EHDS and GDPR, which only time will be able to define, in the knowledge that, as Piero Calamandrei wrote, "the articles of law, once out of the mind of the legislator, are like children sent into the world in search of fortune".

4 Conclusion

In conclusion, from a negotiating perspective, one could ask whether the circulation of electronic health data, within the meaning of the new regulation, can also take place by means of contractual structures; i.e. whether the data subject can "hand over" his information in return for some form of remuneration. This opens up the delicate issue of the secondary use of data and the related possibility of remuneration. Interestingly, this issue has been taken into account in Art. 62 of the Regulation with reference to the fees that the bodies responsible for access to health data or the holders of the trustworthy health data referred to in Art. 72 may charge for making electronic health data available for secondary use.

In this framework, the civil law expert cannot help but reflect (not only on the circulation of health data) on the circulation of a further product, a "digital good": namely, the systems of "electronic medical records" (Art. 25 et seq.).

Furthermore, in relation to the phenomenon under consideration, the production of strong economies and exchanges, as well as the constitution of a market and a system of economic-legal relations, is inevitably linked to the ability to regulate both the contents and forms of the operations performed and of the acts and negotiation models in which they are substantiated.

The interpretation of the circulation of such products, also from a contractual perspective, inevitably prompts the question – ultimately – of what the characteristics and components of the relevant negotiation models should be.

In fact, the Regulation, lays down measures to ensure the implementation of a self-certification model for electronic health record systems, aiming to ensure their compatibility across various systems and thereby facilitate the seamless flow of electronic health data in the European context.

In this regard, specific obligations are laid down for each economic operator producing or adopting electronic health record systems. In addition, requirements are introduced regarding the compliance of these systems, as well as the obligations of the market surveillance authorities responsible for electronic health record systems in the context of their market surveillance activities.

Bibliography

1. EU Commission (2022) Study on an infrastructure and data ecosystem supporting the impact assessment of the European Health Data Space. https://health.ec.europa.eu/publications/study-infrastructure-and-data-ecosystem-supporting-impact-assessment-european-health-data-space_en
2. Guarda P (2019) I dati sanitari. In: Cuffaro V, D'Orazio R, Ricciuto V (eds) I dati personali nel diritto europeo. Giappichelli, Torino, pp 591–626
3. Perlingieri C, Cocco A (2024) 'Primary' and 'secondary' use of electronic health data. Ital Law J 10:275–295
4. Ricciuto V (2022) L'equivoco della privacy. Persona vs. dato personale. Edizioni Scientifiche Italiane, Napoli
5. Terzis P, Santamaria Echeverria OE (2023) Interoperability and governance in the European Health Data Space regulation. Med Law Int 23:368–376
6. Viterbo FG (2024) Governance and processing of personal data in the Italian healthcare system in the light of EU principles. Actualidad Jurídica Iberoamericana 20:1052–1087

Chapter 3
Health Data and Scientific Research in the Light of the New European Governance

Francesco Giacomo Viterbo

1 Health Data: From Their Mere Protection and Administration to Their Governance for Medical Research and Public Healthcare Policy

The field of scientific research, especially medical research, is undergoing a transition and approaching a real revolution, particularly in terms of the resources that will be available soon.

One of the essential resources for research is data and, in the field of medical research, "health data". This term seems to refer to personal and non-personal data processed for purposes related to the provision of healthcare—in order to assess, maintain, or restore the state of health of the data subject—or relevant social/administrative services (so-called primary use), as well as for research purposes, other than the initial purposes for which data were collected (so-called secondary use). Health data includes certain special categories of personal data pursuant to Art. 9 of the General Data Protection Regulation (EU Regulation 2016/679, hereinafter: GDPR), namely "data concerning health" as defined in Art. 4(15) of the GDPR and "genetic data" as defined in Art. 4(13) of the GDPR. For genetic data, the law provides for additional precautions, which, however, will not be specifically analysed in this chapter.

The role of health data and the interests associated with it are changing and becoming increasingly central.

Traditionally, this data requires the highest level of protection, as its circulation exposes the individuals to whom it refers to the risk of personal injury. Hence, the

F. G. Viterbo (✉)
University of Salento, Lecce, Italy
e-mail: francesco.viterbo@unisalento.it

A. Bernes, S. Thobani (eds.), *Digitalisation in Health Care between New Technologies, Data and Research*, Services and Business Process Reengineering, https://doi.org/10.1007/978-981-95-6982-3_3

general rule prohibiting processing under Art. 9(1) of the GDPR applies, except where exemptions are provided for in paragraph 2. On the public side, it is well known that in Italy health data are processed by Regional Health Systems and the National Health System (SSN) for purely administrative and expenditure planning purposes, with strict obligations to protect data subjects and unsatisfactory management results. The principles set out in Art. 5 of the GDPR—lawfulness, purpose limitation, data minimisation, accuracy, storage limitation, integrity and confidentiality, and accountability—are an expression of this primary need for data protection.

In recent years, health data has become more than just an asset to be protected and managed. It is also a valuable resource that must be leveraged and governed for the benefit of both the individuals to whom it relates and society.

As regards the first aspect, consider the phenomenon of "precision medicine", which consists of individualising treatment processes through the development of so-called tailored therapy, an emerging therapeutic paradigm aimed at offering the most suitable and appropriate medication to individual patients through the application of targeted interventions based on knowledge of their genetic/molecular profile and individual disease status, in order to predict the likelihood of response to treatment (this includes, for example, CAR-T or Chimeric antigen receptor T cell therapies, which are personalised cancer therapies). At the same time, medicine and biomedical engineering are studying personalised solutions to improve human health, aimed, for example, at compensating for numerous forms of disability or physical impairment with the support of "custom-made device", including implantable or wearable devices. Such devices are intended for the sole use of a particular patient, exclusively to meet their individual conditions and needs, under the definition in Art. 2(3) of Regulation (EU) 2017/745. In this perspective, it is not *Big Data* but *Small Data* (an expression borrowed from a book by Martin Lindstrom) that are of essential importance, i.e. those (personal) data that are immediately capable of enabling the personalisation of a service by adapting it to the uniqueness of the person for whom the service is intended.

As for the second aspect, public interest in the use of health data for research and healthcare public policy governance has grown exponentially following two phenomena that have changed history and brought about a change of course: the COVID-19 pandemic emergency and the risk of new pandemics, on the one hand, and the development of Artificial Intelligence (AI), on the other.

The pandemic has greatly accelerated the 2020 European Data Strategy, i.e. the development and implementation of a health data governance policy based on new principles. It is increasingly recognised that health data generated in different contexts have significant long-term and multifaceted utility, far beyond the specific clinical and diagnostic use for which they were initially collected. In the field of biomedical research, significant efforts are being made to make health data findable, accessible, interoperable, and reusable—in accordance with the principles of Findability, Accessibility, Interoperability, and Reusability (hereinafter: FAIR principles)—with the aim of leveraging different sets of health data isolated in multiple institutions and storage environments. The FAIR principles must be reconciled with the principles of the GDPR.

The development of AI systems with the ability to self-learn, make autonomous decisions, and create innovative outputs, even if sometimes inexplicable by science, has led to a strong push towards the exploitation of personal and non-personal data as raw material for new forms of research and scientific investigation.

2 Secondary Use of Health Data and Scientific Research

Scientific research may be one purpose of health data processing, which usually follows the primary use, i.e. the processing of data for diagnosis, healthcare, or treatment purposes. Contemporary medical and biomedical research relies heavily on the secondary use of personal health data obtained in another clinical or research context.

Under the GDPR, data controllers must comply with the principle of purpose limitation, which limits further processing of personal data beyond the purpose for which the data were initially collected, unless the purpose of the further processing is compatible on the basis of a test to be carried out in accordance with the criteria set out in Art. 6(4). However, Artt. 5(1)(b) and 89 of the GDPR expressly provide that further processing of personal data for scientific research purposes is not considered incompatible with the initial purposes for which the data were collected. Similarly, Recital 50 states that further processing for "scientific or historical research purposes" or statistical purposes "should be considered to be compatible lawful processing operations". These provisions provide grounds for exempting data controllers conducting scientific research from carrying out a compatibility test under Art. 6(4) of the GDPR for further processing.

However, this should not be misunderstood to mean that the processing of personal data for scientific research purposes is automatically permitted.

Firstly, the definition of "scientific research" within the meaning of the GDPR is highly debated. Recital 159 partly incorporates the statement made by the European Data Protection Supervisor (EDPS) in its "Preliminary Opinion on data protection and scientific research" of January 6, 2020, namely that "The GDPR assumes a broad conception of research, including technological development, fundamental and applied research and privately funded research and studies conducted in the public interest in the area of public health". The EDPS also referred to "the principle that genuine research using massive data sets accumulated in the digital economy must be carried out with a public interest aim and within institutional structures for accountability". Therefore, the special data protection regime for scientific research is applicable when, at the same time, (a) personal data are processed; (b) relevant sectoral standards of methodology and ethics apply (medical research is strictly subject to ethical standards and controls); (c) the research is carried out with the aim of growing society's collective knowledge and well-being, as opposed to serving primarily one or several private interests.

Medical and biomedical research is a field of research that differs from others because it draws on health data and encompasses multifaceted realities.

Consider the following two examples. The first is the case of a hospital that performs clinical tests on an individual to diagnose a particular disease and subsequently decides to use the health data collected in an unrelated research study. The case of IRCSS (Istituti di Ricovero e Cura a Carattere Scientifico) is different, as, according to Art. 110 bis, paragraph 4, of the Legislative Decree No. 196/2003 (hereinafter: Privacy Code), the processing of personal data collected by such Institutes in the course of clinical activities for research purposes does not constitute further processing by third parties, given the instrumental nature of the healthcare activity carried out in relation to the research activities.

3 Legal Basis and Other Conditions for the Lawfulness of Processing Health Data for Research Purposes

Health data relating to an individual are considered highly sensitive, requiring carefully designed safeguards for their responsible use. The processing of such data must meet the dual requirement of having a suitable legal basis under Art. 6 of the GDPR and falling within the cases of exemption from the prohibition on processing provided for in Art. 9(1) of the GDPR.

As regards the legal basis for processing, this can be found in the consent of the data subject pursuant to Art. 6(a); or/and in Art. 6(e), whereby processing is necessary for the performance of a task carried out in the public interest; or/and in Art. 6(f), whereby processing is necessary for the purposes of the legitimate interests pursued by the controller, except where such interests are overridden by the interests or fundamental rights and freedoms of the data subject which require protection of personal data.

With regard to exemptions from the prohibition on processing special categories of data, Art. 9(2)(j) provides for an exception to the prohibition when processing is necessary for scientific research purposes, based on Union or national law, provided that it is proportionate to the aim pursued, provides for suitable and specific measures to safeguard the fundamental rights and the interests of the data subject, and complies with Art. 89(1).

Art. 89(1) provides that processing shall be subject to appropriate safeguards for the rights and freedoms of the data subject. In particular, "technical and organisational measures" shall be implemented "in order to ensure respect for the principle of data minimisation". Where possible, research purposes shall be achieved "by further processing which does not permit or no longer permits the identification of data subjects" or by "pseudonymization, provided that those purposes can be fulfilled in that manner".

It should be noted that the process of anonymising personal data constitutes processing of personal data within the meaning of the GDPR and consists of a technique designed to make it impossible, by reasonably usable means, to re-identify natural persons; however, anonymised data does not fall within the scope of the

GDPR (see recital 26). When pseudonymisation and encryption techniques are applied to personal data, the data are still considered "personal data" within the meaning of the GDPR (see Art. 4(5) of the GDPR). In this regard, it should be noted that the anonymisation of personal data can be difficult to achieve (and maintain) due to the continuous advancement of available technology and progress in the field of re-identification. For this reason, the anonymisation of personal data should be approached with caution in the context of scientific research. This risk, highlighted by the EDPB, is confirmed by the Italian Data Protection Authority's (hereinafter: Garante) decision no. 226 of June 1, 2023. In this case, the complex process put in place by the data controller to eliminate any risk of re-identification of the data of the patients involved was classified as pseudonymisation rather than anonymisation, with significant repercussions.

The "appropriate safeguards" referred to in Art. 89 of the GDPR draws attention to the principle of accountability, which is fundamental in that it requires data controllers to honestly assess and responsibly manage the risks inherent in their research projects. These risks can be very high when, for example, health data is being processed. It is therefore essential to carry out a data protection impact assessment (DPIA), where required under Art. 35 of the GDPR, for the purpose of subsequently configuring and adopting appropriate technical and organisational measures, with an obligation of transparency regarding this assessment.

Among the measures that can be adopted to this end, in addition to anonymisation or pseudonymisation of data, the use of so-called synthetic data and, above all, Federated Learning (FL) are noteworthy in practice. The latter generally consists of a technique for training a Machine Learning (ML) algorithm in decentralised collaborative learning contexts, where the algorithm is trained on multiple local data sets stored in isolated databases (i.e. local nodes) such as smartphones, tablets, and PCs, without the need to collect and process training data in a centralised data server. Only the training results (i.e. the parameters) are exchanged at a certain frequency, which requires a central server to coordinate the training process (centralised FL) to aggregate the training results and calculate the global model. The natural advantage of FL is its ability to comply with GDPR, as personal data is stored and processed locally, and only model parameters are exchanged.

Other legal constraints on medical research may arise from the discretion of EU Member States to introduce additional restrictions on the processing of health and genetic data pursuant to Art. 9(4) of the GDPR. This may represent an obstacle to cross-border European medical research.

In Italy, the further processing of health data for scientific research in the medical, biomedical, and epidemiological fields—in accordance with Art. 110 of the Privacy Code—requires the consent of the data subject after adequate information has been provided, where this is possible and does not involve a disproportionate effort, as is the case, for example, with prospective studies. However, in cases where informing the data subjects and obtaining their consent is impossible, involves a disproportionate effort, or risks compromising the purposes of the research, as is the case for many retrospective observational studies, the data controller must take appropriate measures to protect the rights of the data subjects and submit the research program to the competent local ethics committee for review and, until recently, to the Garante for prior consultation pursuant to Art. 36 of the GDPR. Indeed, this latter obligation, requiring an extremely burdensome procedure, had a negative impact on medical research projects—in particular retrospective ones—and was removed from the first paragraph of Art. 110 (as amended by Art. 44, paragraph 1-bis, of Decree Law No. 2 of March 2, 2024, No. 19, converted, with amendments, by Law No. 56 of April 29, 2024). As a result, it remained in force only between September 2018 and May 1, 2024.

It follows that the data controller, in addition to taking appropriate measures to protect the rights, freedoms, and legitimate interests of the data subject, and obtaining the favourable opinion of the competent ethics committee at the territorial level on the research project, as provided for in Art. 110 of the Code, must also accurately justify and document the existence of ethical or organisational reasons for which informing the data subjects and therefore obtaining their consent is impossible or involves a disproportionate effort; the controller must also carry out and publish the DPIA, in accordance with Art. 35 of the GDPR, and notify the Garante.

A legal basis for processing health data for research purposes may be found under Art. 6(1)(e) and Art. 9(2)(g) of the GDPR when processing is necessary for reasons of substantial public interest, on the basis of Union or Member State law. In Italy, on this legal basis, public entities and private non-profit entities, IRCCS, as well as private entities operating in the healthcare sector within the scope of research projects involving the aforementioned entities, are permitted to make secondary use of personal data, including sensitive data, that has already been collected and does not contain any direct identifying elements (i.e. pseudonymized data), without the need for specific consent, for research and experimentation purposes aimed at developing AI systems in the healthcare sector. In fact, Article 8(1) of Law No. 132/2025, containing *Provisions and delegations to the Government on artificial intelligence*, expressly qualifies such data processing as activities of significant public interest, thus supplementing the provisions of the Regulation (EU) 2024/1689 (AI Act).

4 Additional Issues Relating to the Processing of Personal Data for Medical Research Purposes

Consent as a requirement for the lawfulness of data processing pursuant to Art. 6(1)(a) and Art. 9(2)(a) of the GDPR must be freely given, specific, informed, unambiguous, and explicit where it relates to the processing of special categories of data. It differs conceptually and operationally from the "informed consent" of human participants in research. With regard to the processing of personal data for scientific research purposes, Recital 33 of the GDPR allows for greater flexibility in informing the data subject about the purposes of the research in order to obtain their consent, since in such cases it is not always possible to fully identify the purpose of the processing at the time of data collection. Therefore, it is possible for the data subject to give their consent only to certain areas of research or parts of research projects to the extent allowed by the intended purpose (this is referred to as "broad consent"). In this regard, the EDPB has explained that when research purposes cannot be entirely detailed upfront, the data controller should explore alternative methods to uphold the essence of consent requirements. One such approach could involve allowing individuals to provide consent for a broader research purpose initially, with more specific consent obtained later for individual stages or aspects of the research project. This adopts a phased strategy, where general consent is secured at the outset, followed by detailed consent as the project progresses to specific activities or procedures. In such cases, adequate safeguards should be provided to increase the transparency of the processing during the research project, as well as adequate procedures for withdrawing or further specifying consent.

Further consideration should be given to how the principle referred to in Recital 50 of the GDPR operates in the field of medical research. According to this principle, in the event of further processing of personal data for scientific research purposes, "no legal basis separate from that which allowed the collection of the personal data is required".

This aspect was analysed in depth by the EDPB in Opinion No. 3 of 2019, which deals with Art. 28(2) of Regulation (EU) 536/2014 on clinical trials on medicinal products for human use. This provision refers to situations where the sponsor may wish to process clinical trial data "outside the protocol", but "exclusively for scientific purposes". In such cases, the Regulation provides that consent to the processing of data for this specific purpose must be sought from the data subject at the time of requesting his or her informed consent to participate in the clinical trial. Regarding the legal basis for this further processing of data for research purposes, the following two possibilities can be envisaged:

(a) Consent pursuant to Art. 6(1)(a) of the GDPR is required as a specific legal basis, in addition to that required for the primary purpose of clinical trials
(b) The data controller may subsequently process the data without a new legal basis being required; the presumption of compatibility under Art. 5(1)(b) of the GDPR, subject to the conditions set out in Art. 89, should not be generally excluded for the secondary use of clinical trial data outside the protocol for other scientific purposes.

Well, the same problem of interpretation may arise in Italy for cases where the consent of the data subject is necessary for the processing of health data for medical research purposes, since the conditions set out in Art. 110(1) of the Privacy Code do not apply. In fact, while the consent of the data subject is necessary, Art. 6(4) of the GDPR excludes the compatibility test for further processing for a different purpose when the latter is based on the consent of the data subject. This gives rise to the following two possible scenarios.

Firstly, the secondary use of health data for medical research purposes can be considered, in these cases, not as further data processing for a compatible purpose pursuant to Art. 6(4) of the GDPR, but rather as independent data processing with its own legal basis (consent). Consequently, the use of health data for medical research purposes would effectively mark a "reset" in the data processing chain to the extent that it requires its own legal basis.

In accordance with a different interpretation, despite the need for consent, the secondary use of health data for medical research purposes would fall within the scope of further processing for a compatible purpose under Art. 6(4) of the GDPR, the legal basis for which would be the same as that which allowed the data to be collected. That said, consent to the processing of health data for scientific study would not be a legal basis for processing for research purposes, but rather an additional guarantee under Art. 89 of the GDPR or an additional condition under Art. 9(4) of the GDPR, in a manner similar to that provided for genetic data under Art. 2-septies, paragraph 6, of the Privacy Code. This could be said whenever the research is carried out by the same person who collected the data in accordance with the principle of lawfulness. This interpretation would be consistent with the view of some scholars that the additional conditions and restrictions that may be introduced by the Member States referred to in Art. 9(4) of the GDPR are not relevant to assessing the lawfulness of the data processing.

These legal issues may have significant implications and risk undermining the simplifications and derogations provided for the processing of health data for scientific research purposes.

5 From the "European Data Strategy" to the "European Health Data Space": A New Approach Based on Data Accessibility and Availability in a Secure Processing Environment

It can be said that profound changes are underway in the field of medical research, based primarily on Art. 179(1) of the TFEU and, more recently, on the European Commission Communication of February 19, 2020, entitled "A European Strategy for Data", with which the Union intended to establish a regulatory framework for the governance of "common European data spaces" in strategic sectors and areas of public interest.

Following this strategy, which aims to encourage data sharing and reuse, including for medical research and health policy, the Union adopted Regulation (EU) 2022/868 of May 30, 2022, on European data governance (the so-called Data Governance Act) and Regulation (EU) 2025/327 of February 11, 2025, on the European Health Data Space (hereinafter: EHDS Regulation), which provides for common rules, standards, and infrastructures and a governance framework, with a view to facilitating access to electronic health data for the purposes of primary use of electronic health data and secondary use of those data.

At the heart of this new regulatory framework, there appears to be a fundamental shift in the approach to the issue of data circulation. There is a gradual move away from the idea—central to the GDPR—of data circulation through processing operations, divided into distinct stages based on purpose. In this perspective, each stage of the data life cycle begins when a data controller collects personal data and ends with the achievement of the purposes for which the data controller collected the data (data controller and purpose-centric view). A first sign contrary to this approach is provided for in Art. 99(1) of the Privacy Code, according to which the processing of personal data for scientific research purposes may continue beyond the period necessary to achieve the purposes for which the data were collected and processed.

The Data Governance Act and the EHDS Regulation are increasingly establishing the idea of a continuous flow of data within a space where its entire life cycle takes place, from generation to anonymisation or deletion. It is an approach focused on data and the environment in which it carries out its life cycle.

This approach began to take shape with the possibility that personal data could be made available by the data subject for altruistic and solidarity purposes that were not necessarily predetermined.

The principle of "data altruism" has been implemented in the Data Governance Act, which encourages the voluntary sharing of data on the basis of consent given by data subjects to the processing of personal data concerning them for purposes of general interest, including scientific research in the general interest, without requesting or receiving compensation beyond the costs incurred in making the data available. This could help facilitate the voluntary establishment of large-scale data "pools" or "repositories", enabling analysis through algorithmic processes and machine learning. The responsibility for creating and managing these repositories would lie with "Union-recognised data altruism organisations", i.e. non-profit entities meeting specific criteria to foster trust and credibility among the public.

An essential driver of data altruism is trust, which is also a consequence of the strategy creating a protected and secure processing environment in which anyone can make even the most sensitive personal data available without particular risk.

The same Regulation defines a "secure processing environment" as "the physical or virtual environment and organisational means to ensure compliance with Union law, such as Regulation (EU) 2016/679, in particular with regard to data subjects' rights, intellectual property rights, and commercial and statistical confidentiality, integrity and accessibility, as well as with applicable national law, and to allow the entity providing the secure processing environment to determine and supervise all data processing actions, including the display, storage, download and export of data and the calculation of derivative data through computational algorithms". However, in the case of processing of personal electronic health data, the secure processing environment shall also comply with the security measures set out in paragraph 1, points (a) to (f), of Art. 73 of the EHDS Regulation.

The concept of "protection" shifts from (personal) data to the processing environment, i.e. the space in which data can begin and continue their life cycle.

Another case of data altruism is the non-exercise of the right to exclude the processing of personal electronic health data for secondary use, as provided for in Art. 71 of the EHDS Regulation. In the context of personal health data, data altruism operates by default, except for the possibility of opting out, according to a mechanism that the EHDS Regulation borrowed from the legal experience of Finland, which was among the first European countries to adopt a law on the secondary use of health data in 2019.

The idea of promoting accessibility, sharing, and reuse of electronic health data is increasingly shaping the organisation of the digital health system through a national infrastructure capable of ensuring the interoperability of clinical data and documents and of interoperating with the information systems used by local health facilities; and, at the supranational level, a dual cross-border infrastructure for primary use (MyHealthData@EU, to which the "digital health authorities" designated by the Member States are connected) and for secondary use of electronic health data (HealthData@EU, to which the "bodies responsible for access to health data" designated by the Member States are connected).

The MyHealthData@EU and HealthData@EU infrastructures, specifically governed by the EHDS Regulation, do not aim to establish one or more central EU databases of health data, but only to facilitate access to such data in a "secure processing environment" with a view to giving priority to the concept of bringing questions to data instead of moving them (see Recital 80). This is envisaged primarily in the interests of patients as users of cross-border health services, as well as for the management of requests for cross-border access to health data for secondary use and to enable the linking of the health data with data from other data spaces such as those relating to the environment, agriculture, and social sector.

Recital 61 of the EHDS Regulation states that the secondary use of health data under the EHDS will enable public, private, and not-for-profit entities, as well as individual researchers, to have access to health data for research, innovation, policymaking, educational activities, patient safety, regulatory activities, or personalised medicine. It adds that the provision of data will support activities related to scientific research, interpreting this concept in a broad manner, including technological development and demonstration, fundamental research, applied research, and privately funded research. Activities related to scientific research include innovation activities such as training of AI algorithms that could be used in healthcare or the care of natural persons, as well as the evaluation and further development of existing algorithms and products for such purposes.

The EHDS Regulation will be the reference legal act of the Union on the basis of which personal health data will be shared for scientific research purposes pursuant to Art. 6(1)(*e*) and (*f*) in conjunction with Art. 9(2)(*j*) and (*i*) of the GDPR.

It follows that the principle of free movement of data is accompanied by that of availability and accessibility of (personal and non-personal) data, as values perceived as essential. Furthermore, data can indeed serve as a valuable resource with the potential to generate financial benefits. However, certain types of data are gaining increasing social value and importance due to their secondary uses. These uses, aimed at advancing research, improving policies, and enhancing services, position such data as a crucial resource for fostering community well-being.

In the context of health data, the principles of availability and accessibility hold greater significance when compared to the attributes of circulation and the (presumed) patrimonial value. These latter aspects, however, appear to be more characteristic of non-personal data or, at most, personal data that does not fall under the special categories outlined in Article 9 of the GDPR.

Addressing the challenges associated with both the primary and secondary use of electronic health data requires significant effort, particularly from supervisory authorities, to uphold compliance with GDPR principles in this evolving landscape. A key priority is ensuring that EU fundamental rights remain at the heart of the digital transformation, leveraging a human-centric approach to tackle the new issues arising from societal demands for data sharing and increased availability.

Bibliography

1. Amram D (2020) Building up the "Accountable Ulysses" model. The impact of GDPR and national implementations, ethics, and health-data research: comparative remarks. Comput Law Secur Rev 37:1–7
2. Becker R, Chokoshvili D, Comandé G, Dove E, Hall A, Mitchell C, Molnar-Gabor F, Nicolás P, Tervo S, Thorogood A (2022) Secondary use of personal health data: when is it 'further processing' under the GDPR, and what are the implications for data controllers? Preprint at: https://ssrn.com/abstract=4070716
3. Bernes A (2020) La protezione dei dati personali nell'attività di ricerca scientifica. Nuove leggi civili commentate 1:175–205
4. Bolognini L, Zipponi S (2024) Privacy e diritto dei dati sanitari. Giuffrè, Milano
5. Bygrave LA, Docksey C, Drechsler L, Kuner C (eds) (2020) The EU general data protection regulation (GDPR). A commentary. Oxford University Press
6. Camardi C (2023) Sulla Governance digitale europea: una proposta di confronto. Accademia 1:7–10
7. EDPS (2020) Study on the secondary use of personal data in the context of scientific research. Final Report. https://www.edpb.europa.eu/our-work-tools/our-documents/other/study-secondary-use-personal-data-context-scientific-research_en
8. EU Commission (2022) Study on an infrastructure and data ecosystem supporting the impact assessment of the European Health Data Space. https://health.ec.europa.eu/publications/study-infrastructure-and-data-ecosystem-supporting-impact-assessment-european-health-data-space_en
9. EU Commission (2021) Assessment of the EU member states' rules on health data in the light of GDPR. http://ec.europa.eu/dgs/health_food-safety/index_en.htm
10. Guarda P (2019) I dati sanitari. In: Cuffaro V, D'Orazio R, Ricciuto V (eds) I dati personali nel diritto europeo. Giappichelli, Torino, pp 591–626
11. Ienca M, Scheibner J, Ferreti A, Gille F, Amann J, Sleigh J, Blasimme A, Vayena E (2019) How the general data protection regulation changes the rules for scientific research. Study for the European Parliament panel for the future of science and technology. Brussels. http://www.europarl.europa.eu/thinktank/en/document.html?reference=EPRSSTU(2019)634447
12. Perlingieri C (2021) eHealth and data. In: Senigaglia R, Irti C, Bernes A (eds) Privacy and data protection in software services. Springer, pp 127–139
13. Pizzetti F (2021) La Parte I del Codice novellato. In: Id. (ed) Protezione dei dati personali in Italia tra GDPR e Codice novellato. Giappichelli, Torino, pp 74–157
14. Rapisarda I (2021) Ricerca scientifica e circolazione dei dati personali. Verso il definitivo superamento del paradigma privatistico? Eur Dirit Priv 2:301–347
15. Sborlini D (2024) Il broad consent come mezzo per la valorizzazione dei dati personali nell'ambito della ricerca scientifica e il suo rilievo negli spazi di condivisione dei dati. Contratto e impresa 1:223–262

16. Verhenneman G, Claes K, Derèze JJ, Herijgers P, Mathieu C, Rezda R, Vanautgarden M (2019) How GDPR enhances transparency and fosters pseudonymisation. Eur J Health Law 27(1):35–57. https://doi.org/10.1163/15718093-12251009
17. Viterbo FG (2024) *Intuitus personae* e negozi "su misura". Edizioni Scientifiche Italiane, Napoli
18. Viterbo FG (2024) Governance and processing of personal data in the Italian healthcare system in the light of EU principles. Actualidad Jurídica Iberoamericana 20:1052–1087

Chapter 4
Secondary Use of Health Data, Scientific Research, and Experience of the Italian Data Protection Authority

Chiara Di Somma

1 Introduction

Technological progress, data digitisation, and the growing need—if not urgency—of the scientific community to make greater use of health data for research purposes are distinctive features of contemporary society. These developments call for a reassessment of the mechanisms needed to ensure a fair balance between the right to health and the freedom of scientific research, on the one hand, and the rights to data protection and privacy, on the other.

To this end, it is necessary to reason both *de iure condito*, by analysing the rationale and interpretation of the (new) applicable provisions, and *de iure condendo*, by contributing—through legal debate—to future standardisation.

Indeed, the regulatory instruments that constitute, or will constitute, the legal basis for the processing of health data collected or generated in clinical settings and intended for further processing for medical research purposes represent the primary context in which such balancing begins to concretely take shape.

The purpose of this paper is to present and analyse the main regulatory instruments within the Italian and European legal frameworks that may provide a legal basis for the processing of health data for medical research purposes.

This contribution is written in a personal capacity; the views and opinions expressed herein are solely those of the author.

C. Di Somma (✉)
Officer at the Italian Data Protection Authority, Rome, Italy
e-mail: c.disomma@gpdp.it

A. Bernes, S. Thobani (eds.), *Digitalisation in Health Care between New Technologies, Data and Research*, Services and Business Process Reengineering, https://doi.org/10.1007/978-981-95-6982-3_4

2 The Legal Bases for the Processing of Health Data for Medical Research Purposes

Pursuant to Regulation 2016/679 on the protection of natural persons with regard to the processing of personal data and on the free movement of such data (GDPR), the principle of the alternativity of legal bases applies.

Data controllers may choose among the different legal grounds listed under Art. 6 of the GDPR, selecting the one most appropriate to the context and purpose of the processing, as there is no hierarchical order among them. Where the processing involves so-called special categories of personal data, commonly referred to as sensitive data—such as data concerning health— controllers must also identify the appropriate exemption from the general prohibition on processing such data, as provided under Art. 9(1) and (2) of the GDPR.

Exemptions to the prohibition on processing health data for medical research purposes, with the exception of consent, are not self-sufficient; they always and necessarily refer to a Union or Member State law, which must comply with specific requirements regarding proportionality, respect for the essence of the right to data protection, and the provision of appropriate and specific safeguards to protect the rights and freedoms of data subjects (Art. 9(2)(g) and (j)).

Of particular relevance for the field of medical research is also Art. 9(4) of the GDPR, which allows Member States to maintain or introduce further conditions, including limitations, with regard to the processing of genetic data, biometric data or health data.

3 Biomedical and Epidemiological Medical Research Under the Italian Privacy Code

Within the normative space assigned to Member States by Art. 9(2)(j) of the GDPR lies Art. 110 of the Italian Personal Data Protection Code (Legislative Decree no. 196 of 30 June 2003, hereinafter "Privacy Code"), which serves as a legal basis for the processing of health data for medical, biomedical, and epidemiological research purposes.

This provision, implicitly recalling the principle of the alternativity of legal bases, outlines three distinct lawful grounds for the processing of health data for research purposes. In brief, these include consent, the existence of a Union or Member State law, and compliance with safeguards set out by the Data Protection Authority when the processing cannot be grounded in either of the first two bases.

Since the issue to be addressed in the present work is the further processing of data, no attention will be given to data subjects' consent, which presupposes that data are collected directly from them.

Art. 110 of the Privacy Code allows the further processing of health data for medical research purposes if such processing is provided for by a Union or Member

State law in accordance with Art. 9(2)(j) of the GDPR. This includes cases where the research is part of a biomedical or healthcare research program established pursuant to Art. 12-*bis* of Legislative Decree no. 502 of 30 December 1992.

In such cases, the rule requires that a Data Protection Impact Assessment (DPIA) must be conducted and published, in accordance with Art. 35 of the GDPR.

Therefore, data controllers are required to conduct a thorough review of relevant national and European legislation in the field of medical research to identify which laws may provide a valid legal basis for the processing of health data for research purposes under Art. 9(2)(j) GDPR and Art. 110 of the Privacy Code.

The Italian Data Protection Authority has deemed that, in addition to Art. 12-*bis* of Legislative Decree no. 502/1992, Art. 110-*bis*, paragraph 4, of the Privacy Code also falls within the legal framework established under Art. 110, for the portion in question. This provision constitutes the legal basis for the processing of health data for medical research purposes by Scientific Institutes for Research, Hospitalisation and Healthcare (IRCCS), when such institutions originally collected the data in the course of clinical activity.

In this regard, on 6 May 2024, the Data Protection Authority published specific FAQs titled *Legal Bases and Main Requirements for the Processing by IRCCS of Personal Data Collected for Healthcare Purposes for Further Research Purposes* (doc. web. n. 10024215).

It is now necessary to dwell on the third part of Art. 110, paragraph 1, of the Privacy Code, which—as is well known—prior to the amendment introduced in 2024, provided that when it was not possible, due to ethical or organisational reasons, to obtain data subjects' consent for the performance of studies in the medical, biomedical and epidemiological fields, the data controller or study sponsor was required to submit a request for prior consultation to the Data Protection Authority pursuant to Art. 36 GDPR and to obtain the favourable opinion of the competent ethics committee.

This requirement was not consistently observed by all actors in the field and those who complied with it often viewed it as an (additional) obstacle to the timely execution of their studies.

However, the provision enabled the Data Protection Authority to issue numerous decisions offering valuable guidance on the proper processing of data in research contexts. The Authority addressed the lawfulness of processing, the proper designation of data controllers and processors among the various parties involved in research studies, obligations regarding transparency (including the regulation of so-called incidental findings), and data minimisation measures, particularly through pseudonymisation techniques. On the other hand, these decisions gave stakeholders time and opportunity to enhance their expertise and awareness, gradually adopting a more responsible and informed approach to the complex requirements of data protection law.

Art. 44 (1-*bis*) of Decree-Law no. 19 of 2 March 2024, converted with amendments by Law no. 56 of 29 April 2024, introduced a significant change to Art. 110 of the Privacy Code, repealing the requirement for prior consultation in cases where, for the purpose of conducting retrospective studies, it is not possible to obtain the consent of the data subjects, while leaving unchanged the requirement to obtain the opinion of the competent ethics committee. However, the task of identifying additional safeguards to be applied in such cases has been assigned to the Data Protection Authority, pursuant to Art. 106(2)(d) of the Privacy Code.

In its resolution of 9 May 2024, the Authority laid down the safeguards to be implemented where, due to specific ethical or organisational circumstances, obtaining consent from the data subjects is not feasible. In particular, it requires that data controllers:

- Provide a reasoned justification in the research protocol
- Conduct a mandatory Data Protection Impact Assessment (DPIA) pursuant to Art. 35 of the GDPR
- Publish the DPIA—at least in summary form
- Notify the Authority that the above obligations have been fulfilled, specifying the website where the related documentation can be accessed

From a formal perspective, the legislative amendment aligns with prior simplifications introduced into the Privacy Code, particularly those aimed at addressing regulatory gaps in data flows or necessary disclosures. One example is Art. 2-*ter* of the Code, which now requires that, for communications of non-sensitive personal data not explicitly provided for by a legal act, the Data Protection Authority merely be notified at least 10 days before the initiation of such communication or dissemination.

The requirement to carry out and publish a Data Protection Impact Assessment (DPIA) already applies to all processing of "sensitive" data for research purposes when conducted pursuant to a specific legal provision. Where no such legal basis exists, the Authority has additionally imposed the obligation to notify the processing. The rationale for these safeguards lies in reinforcing the principles of accountability and transparency, which have become increasingly central, especially to counteract the opacity of algorithms that are now frequently used in medical research.

The legislative reform mentioned above also enables the Data Protection Authority to assert its role in the medical research sector, not only as an *ex post* supervisory body, but also as an *ex ante* promoter of legal awareness regarding data protection law.

Finally, it is worth emphasising that this simplification for data controllers does not in any way amount to a diminution of protection for data subjects. Rather, it represents a recalibration of the balance between personal data protection and the freedom of scientific research (Art. 9 of the Italian Constitution). This new balance is made possible—and proportionate—because, on the one hand, controllers have shown increased awareness and competence regarding their obligations, and on the other hand, because of the enhanced accountability and transparency measures now in place.

The next step must be the full realisation of accountability, with the hope that stakeholders will adopt a proactive approach, potentially through codes of conduct and certification mechanisms pursuant to Art. 40 et seq. of the GDPR.

Since Art. 106 of the Privacy Code assigns the Data Protection Authority the task of promoting the adoption of Codes of Ethics in the field of research—by specifying in detail the categories of processing activities for which regulation through such codes is encouraged—the Authority, in its resolution of 9 May 2024, has also launched the process of reviewing the Deontological Rules for the processing of personal data for statistical or scientific research purposes, pursuant to Art. 2-*quarter* and 106 of the Code.

These rules, which will be legally binding and whose violation will result in administrative sanctions, will apply to both statistics and research, across the board, and not just to medical research. The new framework will provide an opportunity to:

- Complete the relevant sectoral legislation
- Fill existing regulatory gaps
- Clarify controversial issues
- Identify additional safeguards where necessary.

4 Registers and Research Conducted in the Public Interest

Art. 110 of the Privacy Code, as analysed above, serves as an exceptional and alternative legal basis to consent, a sort of fallback provision. However, several other legal bases authorise the further processing of data for research purposes, including biomedical and epidemiological research.

Recital 157 of the GDPR highlights the importance of "registers" as single-issue databases that are extremely useful for epidemiological research and predictive analysis, enabling future trends and developments in specific pathologies to be inferred by studying their historical patterns.

Italian law already provides a well-developed framework for disease surveillance systems and pathology registers, as set out in Art. 12, paragraphs 10 to 14, of Decree-Law no. 179 of 18 October 2012, and the Ministerial Decree of 3 March 2017, along with related implementing decrees on which the Data Protection Authority is required to provide its opinion.

Also relevant is the legislation governing official statistics, namely Legislative Decree no. 322 of 1989. The National Statistical Programme has long included epidemiological studies, particularly those conducted by the National Institute of Health and the Ministry of Health.

It is also important to mention Legislative Decree no. 33 of 2013, Art. 5-*ter*, which establishes the legal basis allowing researchers—including those conducting statistical research outside the National Statistical System—to collect or access official statistical data.

Interestingly, the regulation of access has been delegated in its operational details to the Guidelines for Scientific Access to Elementary Data of the National Statistical System (SISTAN), adopted by the ComStat (the Steering Committee for Statistical Information), on which the Data Protection Authority issued an opinion dated 21

June 2018. These guidelines stipulate that ISTAT data, derived from the databases of both public and private entities, may be accessed subject to the adoption of robust pseudonymisation techniques, or alternatively, may be processed within secure processing environments.

5 Evolving Legal Framework in the Italian Context

Scientific research—including medical research—may require the combination (as Recital 157 of the GDPR puts it, "coupling" in the original English version) of information contained in registers, understood as databases, also with a view to conducting studies on larger population groups (again, citing Recital 157 of the GDPR).

In this regard, attention should be drawn to paragraphs 1-*bis* and 1-*ter* of Art. 2-*sexies* of the Privacy Code, introduced, respectively, by Art. 9(1)(b)(2) of Decree-Law no. 139 of 8 October 2021, converted with amendments by Law no. 205 of 3 December 2021, and Art. 44(1)(a)(2) of Decree-Law no. 19 of 2 March 2024, converted with amendments by Law no. 56 of 29 April 2024.

These provisions foresee that pseudonymised health data held by the Ministry of Health, the National Institute of Health (ISS), by the National Agency for Regional Health Services, the Italian Medicines Agency, the National Institute for Health, Migration and Poverty, and the Autonomous Regions and Provinces, may be interconnected by ministerial decree—issued after consulting the Data Protection Authority—for the pursuit of their institutional objectives (Art. 2-sexies, para. 1-*bis*); a national-level interconnection of individual-based health information systems, including the Electronic Health Record (EHR or Fascicolo Sanitario Elettronico FSE), or other public administration databases, may be implemented. A secure processing environment must be established in which anonymised or pseudonymised data will be made available for institutional purposes (Art. 2-*sexies*, para. 1-*ter*).

Where research falls within the institutional purposes of the entities involved in such interconnections, those entities may rely on the above legal provisions as the legal basis for processing health data already held by other public administrations—subject, of course, to the limits and conditions outlined in implementing regulations in line with the principle of proportionality.

6 The Electronic Health Record (EHR)

Art. 2-sexies also provides an opportunity to focus on the Electronic Health Record, which is expected to become a crucial source of real-world data for research.

The EHR has always been an instrument theoretically suitable for use in medical, biomedical and epidemiological research (see Art. 12(2)(b) of Decree-Law no. 179

of 18 October 2012, converted with amendments by Law no. 221 of 17 December 2012, as amended).

Ministerial Decree of 7 September 2023—commonly referred to as "FSE 2.0"—updated the framework governing the FSE and referred the use of its data for research purposes to future decrees.

A first significant milestone was achieved with the Ministerial Decree of 31 December 2024, which established the Health Data Ecosystem (*Ecosistema di Dati Sanitari*—EDS) under Art. 12(15-quater) of Decree-Law no. 179 of 2012.

The EDS is a data ecosystem designed to enable service delivery through the use of data contained in the EHR, which is progressively incorporated. Among the services offered is the ability to allow institutions and entities statutorily or institutionally authorised to conduct research to process FSE-derived data within the EDS for research purposes.

Art. 17 of that decree provides that, for scientific research in the medical, biomedical and epidemiological fields, the EDS shall make available data extraction services for anonymised data, where applicable, via AGENAS (the National Agency for Regional Health Services). Moreover, paragraph 4 of Art. 17 states: "A subsequent decree shall establish specific provisions for the activation of EDS services enabling the processing of personal data for the purposes of study and scientific research in the medical, biomedical, and epidemiological fields, in compliance with the safeguards provided for under Article 89 of the GDPR" (T.a).

7 European Health Data Space: Regulation (EU) 2025/327

At the European level, particular attention must be paid to the recent establishment of the European Health Data Space (EHDS)—the first common European data space dedicated to a specific sector, in line with the EU data strategy. It is governed by Regulation 2025/327, dated 11 February 2025.

The EHDS constitutes a comprehensive and complex set of legal and technical rules designed to facilitate individuals' access to and control over their electronic health data while also promoting its interoperable reuse for purposes of public interest, including scientific research.

The EHDS aims to:

- Enable individuals to access, control and share their electronic health data across borders to support the provision of healthcare (primary use of data);
- Enable the secure and trustworthy reuse of electronic health data in areas such as research, innovation, policy-making and regulatory activities (secondary use of data);
- Promote a single market for electronic health record systems to support both primary and secondary data uses.

Under the EHDS Regulation, the term "secondary use of data" refers to "The processing of electronic health data for the purposes set out in Chapter IV of this

Regulation, which are different from the original purposes for which such data were collected or produced" (Art. 2(1)(e)).

The types of electronic health data eligible for secondary use are listed in Art. 51(1) of the EHDS Regulation. Subsequent paragraphs of that article allow individual Member States to make adjustments, including: adding other categories of electronic health data for secondary use; introducing further conditions for the processing of certain types of data considered particularly sensitive (Art. 51(4)).

As previously noted, secondary use is only permitted where it serves specific purposes set out in Art. 53, among which medical and statistical research are expressly included (paragraph 1, letters c and e).

Art. 55 et seq. of the Regulation define the governance structure and operational mechanisms of secondary data use.

A key role is played by the so-called Health Data Access Bodies, which act as intermediaries between data users (i.e. those requesting access) and data holders. These bodies are entrusted with several tasks, including granting access to data; providing actual access through secure processing environments; preparing and compiling data at the request of the data holders; and pseudonymising or anonymising data (Art. 57).

By operating within the normative frameworks established by Art. 9(2) of the GDPR—particularly subparagraphs (g), (i), and (j)—the EHDS Regulation serves as the legal basis that allows data holders to enable the sharing of electronic health data through these intermediary organisations (Recital 52 of the EHDS Regulation).

However, data users must, in turn, possess a valid legal basis for accessing such information, which must be verified by the Health Data Access Bodies (Recital 52 and Art. 58(1)(a)).

To ensure effective implementation of individuals' right to informational self-determination, the Regulation introduces a "*right to opt-out*" of secondary data use (Art. 71), allowing individuals to exclude their electronic health data from processing for secondary purposes.

Relevant in this context is also the Data Governance Act (Regulation 2022/868), which, while fully respecting the rules on personal data protection, sets out provisions regarding the concept of "data altruism". This is defined as "The voluntary and not-for-remuneration sharing of data based on the consent of the data subject to the processing of their personal data, or the authorization by data holders to allow the use of their non-personal data, for objectives of general interest as laid down in national law, including scientific research in the general interest" (Art. 2(1)(16)) (T.a).

This legal mechanism will only become fully operational when the Agency for Digital Italy (AgID), designated as the competent authority for overseeing the notification procedure for data intermediation services and the registration of data altruism organisations, adopts the necessary technical and organisational measures to support data altruism on the part of controllers, and defines the information to be provided to data subjects regarding the reuse of their data in the public interest (see Art. 2 of Legislative Decree no. 144 of 7 October 2024, in force since 25 October

2024), in addition to fulfilling all other requirements provided under the applicable legal framework (Art. 16-25 of the Data Governance Regulation).

8 Conclusions

The relentless and rapid advancement of technological development, at a pace that is difficult for traditional regulated processes to effectively keep up with, and the consequent new needs of the scientific community require that the legal framework evolve, becoming flexible without being uncertain. It should be defined by primary legislation that sets out principles, which at the same time contain the essential elements of processing and are subsequently developed through implementing acts that can, if necessary, be easily updated.

After conducting the necessary assessment of the need for data, the first line of defence in safeguarding privacy and data protection in the secondary use of data lies in the legislative acts that regulate it.

It is in the regulatory foundation that the principle of proportionality is fulfilled; it is there that the processing finds its legality and fairness; and it is from the regulatory foundation, which must be clear, precise and ensure predictability of the data's fate (Art. 41 GDPR), that data subjects can exercise control over their informations. In cases where data is processed in compliance with a legal obligation, for the performance of a task carried out in the public interest, or collected from third parties, data subjects' right may vary, especially for research purposes. This imposes a strict observance by legislators not only of the GDPR but also of the guidelines provided by the European Data Protection Supervisor and the European Data Protection Board.

In other words, the fair balance between personal data protection and scientific research requires, in a democratic society, precise and stringent evaluations regarding necessity and proportionality, which must be reflected in clear, understandable, and specific legislative acts. Data protection is increasingly a matter of appropriate regulation.

The brief review of relevant national and EU legislation in the field of research shows, in the view of the author that the Member States and the European Union have embarked on the right path. However, it should be emphasised that the search for the right balance is also weighed down by the need for the anticipated solutions to arrive without delay.

Bibliography

1. Italian Data Protection Authority (2023) Decalogue for the realisation of national health services through artificial intelligence systems. Doc. web 9938038
2. Italian Data Protection Authority (2024) FAQ Legal prerequisites and main requirements for the processing by IRCCSs of personal data collected for health care purposes for further research purposes. Doc. web 10024215

3. Italian Data Protection Authority (2024) Resolution promoting the ethics rules for processing for statistical or scientific research purposes pursuant to articles 2-quater and 106 of the code. Doc. web 10016146
4. Italian Data Protection Authority (2023) Opinion on the draft decree of the Ministry of Health, to be adopted with the Minister delegated for technological innovation and digital transition, in agreement with the Minister of Economy and Finance, on the Electronic Health Record (Fascicolo Sanitario Elettronico—FSE). Doc. web 9900433
5. Italian Data Protection Authority (2024) Opinion on the draft decree of the Ministry of Health on the Health Data Ecosystem (EDS), pursuant to Article 12, paragraph 15-quater, of Decree-Law No 179 of 18 October 2012. Doc. web 10062302
6. European Data Protection Supervisor (2017) Necessity toolkit on assessing the necessity of measures that limit the fundamental right to the protection of personal data
7. European Data Protection Supervisor (2019) Guidelines on assessing the proportionality of measures that limit the fundamental rights to privacy and the protection of personal data
8. European Data Protection Supervisor (2024) Guidance for co-legislators on key elements of legislative proposals
9. Di Somma C. (2022) Ricerca scientifica, storica e per finalità statistiche. In: Riccio GM, Scorza G, Belisario E (eds) GDPR e Normativa Privacy, commentario. II ed. Wolters Kluwer, Vicenza, pp 881–904
10. Di Somma C. (2024) Ricerca medica e trattamento dati personali: prime riflessioni sulla modifica dell'art. 110 Codice privacy. https://www.quotidiano-giuridico.it

Chapter 5
Recent Italian Reforms of Health Data Secondary Use Legislation in the Name of Accountability

Luca Bolognini

1 Saying (Temporarily) Goodbye to Accountability in the Medical and Scientific Research Field: The Legislative Step Backwards in Italy, Immediately After the GDPR Application

In accordance with Art. 6(2) of the GDPR, Member States may maintain or introduce more specific provisions to adapt the application of the rules of the GDPR with regard to the processing of data for the fulfilment of legal obligations or for the performance of tasks carried out in the public interest or in the exercise of official authority, determining more precisely specific requirements for processing and other measures to ensure lawful and fair processing, including for other specific processing situations referred to in Chapter IX of the GDPR (including scientific research referred to in Art. 89 of the GDPR). Furthermore, Art. 9(4) of the GDPR allows Member States to maintain or introduce further conditions, including restrictions, with regard to the processing of genetic data, biometric data, or data concerning health.

The Italian legislator therefore took advantage of this opportunity—albeit unfortunately—with Legislative Decree No. 101 of 2018; with this decree, among the various amendments to Legislative Decree No. 196/2003 (the Italian Privacy Code), it introduced a completely unique regime for medical, biomedical, and epidemiological research, amending Art. 110 of the Italian Privacy Code, which is dedicated to this. According to the wording of Art. 110, prior to the intervention of Legislative Decree No. 101/2018, data subject's consent, which constituted the "standard" legal

L. Bolognini (✉)
Italian Institute for Privacy and Data Valorisation, Milan, Italy
e-mail: L.Bolognini@istitutoprivacy.eu

A. Bernes, S. Thobani (eds.), *Digitalisation in Health Care between New Technologies, Data and Research*, Services and Business Process Reengineering, https://doi.org/10.1007/978-981-95-6982-3_5

basis for the processing of data revealing health status for scientific research purposes in the medical, biomedical, or epidemiological field, was not necessary in two specific cases: (1) where the research was provided for by an express provision of law that specifically covered the processing, or was part of a biomedical or health research programme provided for under Art. 12-*bis* of Italian Legislative Decree No. 502 of 30 December 1992 (in which case it was necessary to make a specific notification to the Data Protection Authority, pursuant to the now repealed Art. 39 of the Italian Privacy Code, and wait 45 days, according to a "silence-authorisation" mechanism); (2) when, for particular reasons, it was not possible to inform the data subjects—and therefore obtain their valid consent—and the research programme had been the subject of a reasoned favourable opinion by the competent Ethics Committee at territorial level and had been authorised by the Italian Data Protection Authority ("Garante per la protezione dei dati personali"), also pursuant to the repealed Art. 40 of Italian Privacy Code. The latter article, in particular, provided for the possibility for the Italian Data Protection Authority to resort to "general authorisations" relating to certain categories of data controllers or processing operations. On this basis, over the years, the Data Protection Authority had issued and periodically renewed a series of general authorisations for the processing of data for scientific research purposes, including the processing of data relating to health and sex life and genetic data.

Legislative Decree No. 101/2018, as mentioned, introduced significant changes to the Italian Privacy Code, including the repeal of Art. 40 and the consequent possibility of resorting to general authorisations and confirmed the prevalence of consent as the legal basis for medical, biomedical, and epidemiological research in Italy, while narrowing the scope of exceptions. According to the wording of Art. 110 of the Italian Privacy Code, following the intervention made by Legislative Decree No. 101/2018, the consent of the data subject was not necessary in the following cases: (1) when the research was carried out on the basis of legal provisions (this was, and is, for example, the case of Art. 110-*bis*, par. 4) or regulations or European Union law in accordance with Art. 9(2)(j) of the GDPR, including where the research was part of a biomedical or health research programme provided for in Art. 12-*bis* of Legislative Decree No. 502 of 30 December 1992, and an impact assessment was conducted and made public in accordance with Art. 35 and 36 of the GDPR; (2) where, for specific reasons, informing the data subjects would be impossible or involve a disproportionate effort, or would be likely to render impossible or seriously impair the achievement of the purposes of the research. This could happen, for example, for objective reasons (the data subjects may have died, their contact details may be unknown or very old, they may be in a condition that prevents them from understanding the information, or there may be a large number of data subjects) or for ethical reasons (the data subject may be unaware of their condition). In such cases, the data controller must compensate for the lack of information by taking appropriate measures to protect the rights, freedoms, and legitimate interests of the data subject, and the research programme must be subject to a reasoned favourable opinion from the competent Ethics Committee at the territorial level.

The above rules are still valid and in force. What has changed, as of 1 May 2024, is the last sentence of the first paragraph of Art. 110 of the Italian Privacy Code, as the controversial wording introduced by Legislative Decree No. 101/2018 has been repealed. According to this, between 19 September 2018 and 1 May 2024, research programmes without consent (but not provided for by laws or regulations) also had to be submitted for prior consultation to the Data Protection Authority pursuant to Art. 36 of the GDPR. This prior consultation corresponded to an obligation for the data controllers involved in the research project to request special preliminary authorisation, on a case-by-case basis, from the Data Protection Authority.

It was clear that the 2018 legislation had an unsustainable impact on the regulation of medical, biomedical, and epidemiological research projects, given the impossibility of obtaining consent from data subjects (in particular for retrospective observational studies), as researchers could not rely on general authorisations from the Data Protection Authority and had to resort to ad hoc consultations and authorisations pursuant to Art. 36 of the GDPR.

It should be noted that, between 2018 and 2024, the Italian Data Protection Authority often expressed a favourable opinion on requests for prior consultation, confirming the correctness of the alternative combination of consent and consultation as the legal basis, respectively, for studies where consent could be obtained (prospective studies) and where it was impossible to do so (retrospective studies).

Despite the above and despite the efficient and effective authorisation activity of the Italian Data Protection Authority, there is no doubt that the Italian legislator had in fact complicated and limited the work of researchers and doctors, requiring burdensome procedures (with the associated time and bureaucracy) for research that could previously be carried out on the basis of general authorisations, causing a certain amount of discontent in the world of medical, biomedical, and epidemiological research in Italy, as well as criticism from legal scholars. It is clear, in fact, that the possibility of recourse to general authorisations, based on preventive rules, had the "triple advantage" of reducing the procedural effort for the authority, saving time for the data controller, and ensuring the predictability of the outcome of protection. Paradoxically, the regime of Art. 110 of the Privacy Code in force prior to the 2018 reform was much more consistent and harmonious with the principle of accountability introduced by the GDPR, while the Italian amendment of 2018 moved in the opposite direction and, on closer inspection, was anachronistic.

It should also be noted that the version of Art. 110 approved in 2018 by the Italian legislator did not seem to take into account the favourable regime of the GDPR for scientific research and, on the contrary, by postulating consent as the normal (and main) basis for processing, established an order of priority among the legal bases that was completely opposite to that adopted by Art. 9(2)(j) of the GDPR provides for a basis dedicated to research, while in Art. 110 of the Privacy Code, it is referred to as a mere exception and reiterated by the EDPB in Opinion 3/2019. Moreover, it has been observed that imposing consent as the legal basis at the national level did not appear to be sustainable even on the basis of Art. 9(4) of the GDPR. This provision, in fact, allows Member States to introduce or maintain additional conditions or limitations with regard to the processing of health data, but not to reduce or exclude the legal bases provided for in the GDPR. Furthermore, this approach did not seem to take into account the fact that, in reality, as pointed out in the EDPB opinion, consent should be considered a normally weaker legal basis in these areas, as it is often given by individuals who are emotionally involved and unable to understand its implications, and that, instead of leaving the choice and responsibility to these individuals, the focus should be on protection systems (i.e. security measures), in accordance with Art. 9 and 89 of the GDPR.

The situation in Italy has been exacerbated by the further reduction of the Italian Data Protection Authority's scope of action, as a result of Decree Law No. 139 of 8 October 2021, No. 139, converted with amendments by Law No. 205 of 3 December 2021, which repealed Art. 2-*quinquiesdecies* of the Italian Privacy Code, initially introduced by Legislative Decree No. 101/2018. This article, in fact, regulates processing operations that present high risks for the performance of a task in the public interest and provides, for such operations, the possibility for the Italian Garante, on the basis of the provisions of Art. 36(5) of the GDPR and with general measures adopted ex officio, to prescribe measures and precautions to protect the data subject, to be applied by the data controller. However, the possibility of such general measures was repealed, even though they could have covered, by way of general authorisation, scenarios of scientific research conducted in the public interest.

Until the latest reform of Art. 110 of the Italian Privacy Code, which came into force on 1 May 2024, the rigidity of the negative changes introduced by the legislator of 2018 regarding the legal basis for scientific research in the medical, biomedical, and epidemiological fields seemed insurmountable in Italy. The approach introduced into the regulatory framework by Legislative Decree No. 101/2018 appeared, in fact, excessively conservative and consent-centric, with exceptions that were difficult to achieve or implement in practice, especially in the case of retrospective studies.

2 Two Steps Forward: The 2024 Reform of Article 110, in the Name of Accountability

In January 2024, following several years of work by the Health Working Group as part of the "State of Privacy" initiative of the Italian Data Protection Authority and with the contribution of the Lombardy Life Sciences Cluster and other organisations representing the Italian research community, the reform of Art. 110 of the Italian Privacy Code was finally proposed, as drafted by Luca Bolognini and Diego Fulco. It proposed the elimination of the obligation to consult the Authority in advance and that the Authority could specify the guarantees to be observed in the Rules of Conduct adopted pursuant to Art. 106, par. 2, letter d) of the Italian Privacy Code. With Law No. 56 of 29 April 2024, converting Decree-Law No. 19/2024 (PNRR Decree), the amendment to Art. 110 of the Privacy Code was finally approved and entered into force on 1 May 2024.

There are three considerations in this regard:

- As of 1 May 2024, in Italy, the owners of scientific studies in the medical, biomedical, and epidemiological fields, not covered by laws or regulations and unable to obtain informed consent for the processing of health data from the data subjects, no longer have to request prior consultation/authorisation from the Data Protection Authority;
- The provision for the Italian Authority to identify guarantees to be observed, within the framework of the Rules of Professional Conduct adopted pursuant to Art. 106 and Art. 2-*quater* of the Italian Privacy Code, does not constitute a transition to a general authorisation regime. In fact, neither the identification of such safeguards in the Rules of Professional Conduct nor, indeed, the adoption tout court of the Rules of Professional Conduct (which, in any case, already exist) would constitute an essential precondition for the lawfulness of the processing operations provided for in the first paragraph of Art. 110, as reformulated in 2024
- The clear legislative reference to the fact that the Italian Data Protection Authority directly identifies the safeguards within the Code of Conduct pursuant to Art. 106 and Art. 2-quater of the Italian Privacy Code confirms, in the opinion of the author, the interpretation of these instruments (the Rules of Professional Conduct, in fact) as true expressions of a residual general regulatory power of the Italian Authority, for processing based on compliance with a legal obligation, for the performance of tasks in the public interest or for the exercise of public powers—pursuant to Art. 6(1)(c) and (e) of the GDPR. Although the process of adopting the Rules of Professional Conduct must proceed with the consultation of representative stakeholders of the sectors involved, the initiative for their determination and adoption is now fully attributable to the tasks and powers of the Data Protection Authority. In other words, unlike the Codes of Conduct pursuant to Art. 40 of the GDPR, for the Rules of Conduct pursuant to Art. 2-*quater* of the Italian Privacy Code, the Data Protection Authority will act on its own initiative, while following a procedure with enhanced stakeholder participation.

Finally, it should be noted that, following the amendment to Art. 110, par. 1, third sentence, of the Privacy Code, the final part of the second sentence of the first paragraph of Art. 166 of the Privacy Code, which provided for an administrative fine pursuant to Art. 83(4) of the GDPR for those who did not submit the final part of the second sentence of the first paragraph of Art. 166 of the Privacy Code, which provided for an administrative fine pursuant to Art. 83(4) of the GDPR for those who did not submit "the research programme for prior consultation with the Data Protection Authority in accordance with the third sentence of the aforementioned paragraph" [now repealed, author's note].

By decision of 9 May 2024, the Italian Data Protection Authority, essentially borrowing the contents of the Decision containing the provisions relating to the processing of special categories of data of 5 June 2019, No. 146, pursuant to Art. 21(1) of Legislative Decree No. 101 of 10 August 2018, clarified that ethical reasons—justifying the failure to request consent—are those attributable to the fact that the data subject is unaware of their condition. This category includes research for which the information on data processing to be provided to data subjects would involve the disclosure of information concerning the conduct of the study, knowledge of which could cause material or psychological harm to the data subjects themselves. In the authority's interpretation, organisational impossibility refers to circumstances in which the failure to collect data on the number of data subjects who cannot be contacted to obtain their consent, compared to the total number of subjects to be enrolled in the research, would have significant consequences for the study in terms of the quality of the research results. This is particularly true in view of the inclusion criteria set out in the study, the enrolment procedures, the statistical size of the selected sample, and the length of time that has elapsed since the data relating to the data subjects were originally collected. The Data Protection Authority emphasises that the reasons for organisational impossibility concern both those arising from the circumstance, to be considered entirely residual, that contacting the data subjects would involve a disproportionate effort given the particularly large size of the sample, and those arising from the circumstance, alternative to the previous one, that after every reasonable effort to contact them (including through verification of their status in life, consultation of the data reported in clinical documentation, use of any telephone numbers provided, and acquisition of publicly available contact details) they are deceased or cannot be contacted at the time of enrolment in the study.

In the same provision of 9 May 2024, the authority identified additional safeguards to be observed in cases where it is not possible to obtain the consent of the data subject to process their health data for scientific research purposes in the medical, biomedical, and epidemiological fields. The measures identified are as follows:

(a) In order to respect the principle of accountability, as well as to take appropriate measures to protect the rights, freedoms, and legitimate interests of the data subject, and to obtain the favourable opinion of the competent local ethics committee on the research project, as provided for in Art. 110 of the Italian Privacy Code, the data controller must carefully justify and document, in the research project, the existence of ethical or organisational reasons for which informing the data subjects, and therefore obtaining their consent, is impossible or would involve a disproportionate effort, or would risk making it impossible or seriously compromising the achievement of the research objectives, where appropriate, also documenting the reasonable efforts made to contact them
(b) The data controller must also conduct and publish the data protection impact assessment (DPIA), pursuant to Art. 35 of the GDPR, notifying the Italian Data Protection Authority thereof.

It seems reasonable to interpret provision (b) as meaning that the DPIA may be published on the controller's website even as an abstract, omitting sensitive information or information that could otherwise jeopardise the rights of the parties involved, on the one hand, and the security of data and systems, on the other. In the author's opinion, however, the DPIA should be sent in full to the Data Protection Authority in the communication.

However, in the Author's opinion, it should be underlined that these provisions on the secondary use of health data for scientific research purposes in the medical, biomedical, and epidemiological fields, according to Art. 110, should anyway undergo a necessary review—with a test of regulatory compatibility between Italian law and European regulations—once the EHDS will be fully implemented in Italy.

3 Update Notes on Secondary Use of Sensitive and Health Data for R&D of AI Healthcare Systems: The New Italian Legislation on Artificial Intelligence

In addition to the above, and for the sake of completeness, it is worth mentioning Art. 8 of the new Italian *Law on AI* no. 132/2025: this provision introduced legal bases of substantial public interest for the processing of data, including personal data and special categories of data pursuant to Art. 9(1) GDPR, carried out by public and private non-profit entities, scientific hospitals and research institutes (IRCCS) and private entities operating in the healthcare sector as part of research projects involving public and private non-profit entities or IRCCS, for the purposes of:

1. Scientific research and experimentation in the development of artificial intelligence systems for the prevention, diagnosis, and treatment of diseases, the development of drugs, therapies, and rehabilitation technologies, the creation of medical devices, including prostheses and interfaces between the body and instruments to support the patient's condition, public health, personal safety, health and health safety, as well as the study of physiology, biomechanics, and human biology, including in non-healthcare settings, as necessary for the creation and use of databases and basic models. In terms of accountability, such processing of data must be communicated to the Italian Data Protection Authority, indicating all the information required by Art. 24, 25, 32, and 35 of the GDPR, as well as expressly indicating, where applicable, the subjects identified pursuant to Art. 28 GDPR, and may be initiated 30 days after the aforementioned communication if they have not been subject to a blocking measure ordered by the Data Protection Authority;
2. Data anonymisation or pseudonymisation or creation of synthetic data for the purpose of research and development of artificial intelligence systems in the healthcare sector, as well as for the purposes of planning, managing, controlling, and evaluating healthcare, including the establishment, management, planning, and control of relations between the administration and entities accredited or affiliated with the national health service, as provided for in Art. 2-*sexies*, par. 2, letter v) of the Italian Privacy Code. To help and steer controllers' accountability, the National Agency for Regional Health Services (AGENAS), after consulting the Italian Data Protection Authority, taking into account international standards and the state of the art and technology, may establish and update guidelines for

the procedures for anonymising personal data, and for the creation of synthetic data, including for categories of data and purposes of processing.

In particular, the provisions on the legal basis and guidelines for the data anonymisation or pseudonymisation or creation of synthetic data, for the purposes of research and development of artificial intelligence healthcare systems and for healthcare governance purposes (Sect. 2, above), essentially correspond to the public proposal published by the Italian Institute for Privacy and Data Valorisation in September 2024, which, once again, as was the case for the reform of Art. 110 of the Italian Privacy Code, was taken into account by the legislator.

Bibliography

1. Proposal by the Italian Institute for Privacy and Data Valorisation for the reform of privacy and scientific research. www.istitutoitalianoprivacy.it/2024/01/10/proposta-di-riforma-per-la-privacy-e-la-ricerca-scientifica-tavolo-salute-di-state-of-privacy/
2. Proposal by the Italian Institute for Privacy and Data Valorisation for the introduction, in the Italian law on artificial intelligence, of a legal basis for the data anonymisation or pseudonymisation or creation of synthetic data for the purposes of research and development of AI health systems and health governance. www.istitutoitalianoprivacy.it/2024/09/20/ddl-ai-proposta-iip-una-base-giuridica-per-lanonimizzazione-e-la-sintetizzazione-in-ambito-sanitario/
3. Opinion of the Italian Data Protection Authority (Garante) pursuant to Article 110 of the Code and Article 36 of the Regulation—June 30, 2022, web doc. no. 9791886
4. Opinion of the Italian Data Protection Authority (Garante) pursuant to Article 110 of the Code and Article 36 of the Regulation—July 18, 2023, web doc. no. 9920977
5. Positive decisions issued by the Italian Data Protection Authority (Garante) between 2018 and 2024, prior to the reform of Article 110 (Opinion pursuant to Article 110 of the Code and Article 36 of the Regulation—June 30, 2022, web doc. no. 9791886; Decision of December 10, 2020, web doc. no. 9520597; Decision of October 29, 2020, web doc. no. 9517401; Opinion regarding the processing of personal data, including special categories of data, for medical, biomedical, and epidemiological research purposes, relating to the cohort of patients enrolled in the "MATTERHORN" study—June 20, 2019, web doc. no. 9123447)
6. Bolognini L, Pelino E (eds) (2024) Codice della disciplina privacy, *sub* Art. 110 and Art. 110-*bis*, Milan, Giuffrè Francis Lefebvre

Chapter 6
Challenges and Opportunities in the Evolution of the Italian Electronic Health Record and the Health Data Ecosystem

Alessandra Poggiani

1 Introduction

This article presents a synthetic analysis of the evolving Italian Electronic Health Record (Fascicolo Sanitario Elettronico, FSE) architecture and the newly established Health Data Ecosystem (Ecosistema Dati Sanitari, EDS) within the context of the European Health Data Space (EHDS) framework and how these interconnected initiatives can address longstanding fragmentation in Italy's health data management and healthcare services digitalisation.

Efficient digitisation of healthcare systems demands robust interoperability to ensure seamless data sharing across fragmented and diverse systems. Italy's EHR, Fascicolo Sanitario Elettronico, firstly established with Decree Law 179/2012, exemplifies both the opportunities and complexities of this transition. Despite its potential to gather and unify patients' data across regional health systems, the first Italian EHR has faced persistent hurdles: (a) heterogeneous IT infrastructures, (b) inconsistent adoption of data interoperability standards, and (c) organisational difficulties and resistance. This paper analyses the occurred technical, governance, and regulatory barriers, including unstructured data prevalence, workforce digital literacy gaps, and regional fragmentation. While evaluating these challenges, it illustrates how the current evolutions, aligned with recent European directives objectives, notably the EHDS Regulation, can outline a pathway for an improved and sustainable implementation by adopting solutions grounded in open standards (e.g. HL7 FHIR, openEHR) and federated architectures.

A. Poggiani (✉)
Consorzio CINECA, Bologna, Italy
e-mail: alessandra.poggiani@cineca.it

A. Bernes, S. Thobani (eds.), *Digitalisation in Health Care between New Technologies, Data and Research*, Services and Business Process Reengineering, https://doi.org/10.1007/978-981-95-6982-3_6

The paper specifically describes how the new FSE 2.0 and EDS architectures aim at increasing health care coordination through improved data sharing and access, facilitating access to health data while ensuring data privacy and promoting a patient-centric service delivery model. Early analysis suggests that the synergistic implementation of FSE 2.0 and EDS, if properly aligned with EHDS requirements, can serve as a replicable model for overcoming interoperability barriers in the Italian decentralised healthcare system.

Findings underscore the urgency of data standardisation, infrastructure investments, and professional training to support the potential of the new Italian FSE 2.0 and EDS and their promise of becoming a dynamic platform for interoperable, secure, and ethically compliant health data exchange for medical science and patient care.

2 Lack of Interoperability as a Primary Challenge for Health Data Management

The inhomogeneity of data collection between the various regional health systems in Italy has constituted an obstructing factor against the effective exploitation of health records and data for improving medical assistance and developing data-driven research. The heterogeneity and stratification of the various regional HIS, in fact, combined with the diverse application of legislation on the protection of personal data, lead to significant obstacles in the accessibility and use of health data. Thus, the implementation of interoperability in the health sector is crucial to ensure that clinical information is available and usable when and where needed, supporting informed medical decisions, improving the overall patient experience, and feeding the development of medical research.

However, lack of interoperability, and particularly:

(a) Lack of technological interoperability with regional HISs enabling seamless data exchange: because the infrastructures are regionally based and implemented, EHR data are not stored in a single national centralised cloud environment and do not enable the sharing of data in real time, without the need to extract data through asynchronous and non-dynamic access.
(b) Lack of data interoperability through shared ontologies and standards: health data are often inaccurate and inconsistent, partially because lack of technical standardisation and shared ontologies, but also due to complex and fragmented workflows.

still represents, in Italy (but not only), a gigantic barrier to seizing the full potential of technological data-driven advancement that can dramatically improve healthcare and medical research [11].

Obstacles to data interoperability are not only the result of technological lags or fragmentation among different health authorities and structures but also depend on many different and interlaced reasons. Among them, the multilevel governance of the Italian National Health System, which is reflected in fragmented Information Health Systems among the different regions, and the generally low digital skills and awareness of main actors involved, from nurses to first aid operators and doctors to sector policy makers. Thus, while big data and digitalisation are reshaping and have already changed medical science, the Italian healthcare system governance and healthcare professionals seem not to be fully ready for the challenge.

3 The Italian Context for Health Data Management and the Evolution of Its EHR "Fascicolo Sanitario Elettronico" (FSE) Within the Next Generation EU Italian Plan

Since the early 2000s, Italy has embarked on significant initiatives aimed at transforming and digitally innovating its National Healthcare System (NHS) and its processes. These initiatives initially concentrated on specific functions or domains, such as the digitisation of prescriptions and the introduction of the Health Insurance Card, eventually culminating in the establishment of the Electronic Health Record (hereinafter referred to as "Fascicolo Sanitario Elettronico" or "FSE"). This system was formally introduced under Italian Decree Law no. 179 of 18 October 2012, which was subsequently amended and converted into Law no. 221 of 17 December 2012, serving as a repository for the digital health documents of National Health Service (NHS) patients.

The deployment of the initial version of the Italian Electronic Health Record, FSE, was delegated to the single Regions and Autonomous Provinces, each of which developed its own regional FSE solution tailored to local needs and resources. This decentralised approach, a direct result of the Italian legislative framework, which assigns healthcare management to Regions and Autonomous Provinces, has led to considerable heterogeneity across the country in terms of technological infrastructures, FSE content, and the mechanisms for its access, updating, and dissemination. This heterogeneity has hindered its national effectiveness and concrete benefits for patients, doctors, and medical researchers.

The necessity for a content-uniform, real-time, standardised, and nationally pervasive FSE has become increasingly urgent in the aftermath of the SARS-CoV-2 pandemic [12]. The pandemic health crisis has highlighted the structural challenges within the Italian healthcare system, notably the absence of a unified and interoperable national digital infrastructure capable of delivering reliable and real-time health data promptly for emergency response, continuity of care, and healthcare governance at both national and local levels. The pandemic has unequivocally highlighted the paramount importance of the availability and quality of health data, which is essential not only for delivering optimal healthcare to all patients within the National Health Service (NHS) but also for the development and implementation of effective public health policies based on data-driven research and for ensuring the overall resilience of the healthcare system.

In response to these critical challenges, the Italian National Recovery and Resilience Plan has outlined, within the framework of the EU Next Generation funding programme (Italy Plan—Mission 6—Health), a comprehensive and transformative digitalisation project for the National Health Information System. This initiative aims at designing and implementing a new national Electronic Health Record (Fascicolo Sanitario Elettronico—FSE 2.0[1]) to overcome the previous version's difficulties and its fragmented outcome. Concurrently, there has been a significant renewal of digital health policies at the European level, culminating in a regulation on the European Health Data Space (EHDS),[2] which finally entered into force last March 2025. The EHDS signifies the inaugural sector-specific common data space to be developed under the "European Data Strategy". It seeks to foster shared governance, cross-border portability of health data, and full interoperability among the health systems of EU Member States.

Thus, the current scenario is characterised by a dual digital transition at both the national (FSE 2.0) and the European (EHDS) levels, aimed at establishing a digital health ecosystem predicated on reliable, accessible, interoperable, and secure data sharing. Within this context, the initiatives undertaken at the Italian national level for the implementation of a new version of EHR, namely FSE 2.0, in combination with a Health Data Ecosystem space, seem well-positioned and potentially positive. They not only address the relevant hindrances that became evident in the first Italian EHR phase, the FSE 1.0, such as the lack of a homogeneous EHR standard with structured data and documents distributed nationwide, but they also represent an opportunity to align with the European framework and leverage health data as a strategic asset for the future of public health.

4 The New Italian EHR: Fascicolo Sanitario 2.0

The new Italian Electronic Health Record (EHR), called Fascicolo Sanitario 2.0, represents the pivotal instrument in addressing the challenges associated with health data access and management within the country. The new FSE 2.0 revised federated architecture functions on two levels: 1) Regions and Autonomous Provinces maintain their local systems using shared open standards in a federated network; 2) through data centralisation, it aims at facilitating patients' data collection and storage on a unified platform, thereby ensuring uniform data accessibility nationwide.

A fundamental component of this system is standardisation: the FSE 2.0 endorses the use of shared formats and languages for data recording and exchange. Such

[1] See Decree of the Minister of Health of 7 September 2023 "Electronic Health Record 2.0".

[2] Regulation of the European Parliament and of the Council on the European Health Data Space and amending Directive 2011/24/EU and Regulation (EU) 2024/2847

harmonisation is crucial for ensuring that information is comprehensible and usable across all health information systems, thereby fostering interoperability among the different regional healthcare entities. Another significant improvement that the FSE 2.0 intends to bring is increased accessibility. It should enable healthcare professionals, including physicians and researchers, to swiftly and securely access patients' medical histories, encompassing diagnostic reports, prescriptions, and historical treatments. This accessibility enhances the quality of clinical decision-making and expedites research processes.

Furthermore, the FSE 2.0 architecture integrates data from diverse sources, such as hospitals, outpatient clinics, pharmacies, and laboratories, offering a comprehensive and current perspective on a patient's health status. This capability to aggregate and anonymise data permits the conduct of large-scale clinical and epidemiological studies, contributing to therapeutic innovations and more effective health policy formulation. The implementation of the FSE 2.0 intends to solve the problematic predominant issue of unstructured data, such as PDF documents and textual reports, which currently hinders the automation and advanced analysis of clinical information. At the same time, it addresses the issue of integrating existing healthcare information systems, which are often outdated or heterogeneous, with an advanced standardisation process. To address these critical issues, FSE 2.0. adopts open standards that facilitate system interoperability, such as HL7 FHIR (Fast Healthcare Interoperability Resources) to promote greater consistency and compatibility among different platforms.

The effective implementation of the new FSE 2.0 constitutes one of the most significant challenges in the digital transformation of the Italian National Healthcare System. The critical issues identified thus far with the previous FSE, including data fragmentation, the predominance of unstructured information, and the heterogeneity of information systems, necessitate strategies grounded in open standards, interoperable architectures, and participatory governance models, at least in the management of Information Systems. In this context, the openEHR standard emerges as one of the most promising solutions. OpenEHR is an open specification designed for modelling, storing, and exchanging clinical data, characterised by a clear distinction between the reference model (which defines the technical structures of the data) and the Archetypes layer (which articulates clinical concepts according to a computable logic). This two-layer paradigm allows for a complete separation between content and technological structure, rendering semantic clinical data independent of software platforms, thereby ensuring semantic persistence and long-term reusability. This approach facilitates the integration of heterogeneous systems and enables the development of "open platform" healthcare environments, in which native and computable data can be shared, interpreted, and reused without any loss of clinical meaning.

The new Italian FSE 2.0 implementation project is divided into 3 cohesive and complementary actions:

1. Workstream 1—Creation of a new national architecture for the FSE system to ensure the indexing and standardisation at regional and national level of clinical

documents produced in healthcare facilities and the creation of a national health data ecosystem (EDS) and associated "data-based" services, which meet the needs of citizens (e.g. search and consultation of clinical data, booking and payment of healthcare services, patient empowerment), healthcare professionals (e.g. search and consultation of clinical data of patients for their analysis aimed at supporting clinical decisions in the execution of diagnosis and treatment activities, preventive evaluation of the appropriateness of prescriptions, etc.), Ministry of Health and Regional Health Directorates (to support prevention activities, health planning, and international prophylaxis), and research bodies (to support research activities in the medical and biomedical field)

2. Workstream 2—Technological adaptation at a regional level of the systems producing the minimum clinical data and documents which will feed, in a structured manner and according to interoperability standards defined at a national level, the new FSE 2.0 (e.g. Electronic Medical Records of Wards and Emergency Departments, laboratory and/or outpatient specialist reporting systems) including the systems used by General Practitioners (GPs) and Pediatricians of Free Choice (PFCs), in compliance with the new ESF system architecture defined at a national level (e.g. production of clinical documents with structured and codified data in compliance with HL7-CDA2 standards, adoption of the PaDES digital signature)
3. Workstream 3—Training and engagement by the 21 Regions and Autonomous Provinces of the Healthcare Professionals "called" to feed and consult the new FSE 2.0, through the activation of multi-disciplinary training programmes implemented at a regional level and functional to (1) concretely increase the digital skills of Health Care Professionals in primary care and health (hospital and territorial) and socio-health care; (2) maximise the degree of dissemination, supply, use, and consultation of the ESF 2.0 in every sphere of health care (hospital, territory, primary care, etc.).

5 From Repository to Platform: The Evolution of FSE 2.0 and EDS Through Interoperability Standards

The new FSE 2.0 is conceived not only as a uniform and interoperable collection of digital clinical documents, but as a data-enabled intelligent platform. This transformation is made possible by the simultaneous activation of a complementary and integrated infrastructure: the Health Data Ecosystem (in Italian: Ecosistema Dati Sanitari—"EDS"[3]), an advanced digital infrastructure being designed and implemented under the coordination of the Ministry of Health and the Government Department of Digital Transformation (Implementing Parties of the NGEU—FSE

[3] Decree of the Ministry of Health of 31 December 2024 on the Establishment of the Health Data Ecosystem

project) to collect, integrate, and analyse, in full compliance with current data privacy regulations (European GDPR), health data, and information coming from different sources, and primarily from the new FSE 2.0, with the aim of improving the quality and efficiency of health services provided throughout the country.

Thanks to the data collected through the new FSE 2.0, the EDS intends to pursue the following strategic aims:

(a) Care and prevention: to provide health professionals with "data-driven" services with up-to-date information for accurate diagnosis and timely treatment of individual patients
(b) Study and scientific research: supporting medical research through access to aggregated and anonymised data
(c) Health planning: facilitating the planning and evaluation of health services to improve the efficiency of the NHS
(d) International prophylaxis: managing and monitoring preventive measures against the global spread of diseases.

Combined with EDS, the new FSE 2.0 is therefore designed to be not only a repository of data, but a dynamic and enabling system, designed to generate continuous information value from the data collected from FSE and other public national information systems (e.g. TS, ANA, regional registries).

The transition from static repositories to dynamic platforms represents a crucial evolution in the Italian digital health infrastructure. The Fascicolo Sanitario Elettronico 2.0 (FSE 2.0) and the Ecosistema Dati Sanitari (EDS) exemplify this shift, offering—on paper—a potentially robust framework for semantic and technical interoperability across Italy's healthcare system. Unlike traditional repositories, which have served as passive archives, these new systems are natively aimed at functioning as active platforms in order to facilitate real-time data exchange among all stakeholders including patients, healthcare providers, researchers, and public administrations.

To ensure efficacy, FSE 2.0 and EDS will have to adhere to rigorous functional and non-functional requirements, including:

(a) Interoperability standards: Adoption of international protocols (e.g. HL7 FHIR, openEHR) to harmonise data exchange
(b) Identity and access management: Unambiguous patient and document identification to prevent errors
(c) Consent mechanisms: Real-time electronic informed consent aligned with GDPR (Regulation (EU) 2016/679)
(d) Security-by-design: Multilayered encryption, pseudonymization, and audit trails to safeguard data integrity (ISO/IEC 27001)

Additionally, to be effective, the EDS deployment will need to leverage a systemic approach, balancing interoperability, privacy, and sustainability to promote the new FSE 2.0 potential as a patient-centric and data-driven healthcare enabler. User trust hinges on transparency in data processing, accountability measures, and patient empowerment tools (e.g. granular access controls).

6 Beyond the Technological Architectural Solutions: Organisational Challenges

The sole adoption of more advanced technological standards and platforms will however be insufficient for the successful implementation of the new FSE 2.0 and EDS and a real digitalisation of the Italian national Health System. Healthcare professionals must be actively involved from the initial stages of their implementation, since the experience of end-users is crucial in shaping solutions that can effectively be applied in everyday clinical practice. Their involvement is necessary to enhance healthcare operators' confidence in new technologies, mitigate resistance to change, and promote the active adoption of the new FSE 2.0, ultimately leading to tangible improvements in the quality and safety of healthcare nationwide.

Continuous training of healthcare personnel is also indispensable for the effective implementation of the new technological architectures. Such training must be envisioned as an ongoing process, one that evolves in tandem with technological and regulatory advancements. The introduction of information technology in healthcare has often been perceived as disruptive to the medical sector workforce and their established workflows, potentially increasing administrative burdens and diminishing the time available for direct patient care. This negative perception, frequently exacerbated by past experiences and prejudices stemming from previous unsuccessful implementations (including the FSE 1.0), can lead to disengagement or even active resistance, thereby jeopardising the successful deployment of the new FSE 2.0.

To effectively address these organisational barriers, it will be essential to employ structured change management strategies that integrate training, communication, and ongoing support. Investment in professional training is crucial and should be approached not merely as a transfer of technical skills, but as a comprehensive process that builds awareness of the clinical, organisational, and systemic benefits associated with the use of the FSE 2.0 and EDS. Initiatives aimed at fostering an organisational culture oriented towards innovation and continuous learning are vital to transforming digitisation from a bureaucratic requirement into a strategic tool for enhancing care quality. Valuing end-user feedback, ensuring the adaptability of technological solutions to local contexts, and the presence of clinical leadership actively promoting change represent additional critical success factors. Only healthcare workers who are adequately trained can make informed and valuable use of the capabilities offered by the FSE, thereby contributing to the improvement of clinical processes, information management, and ultimately, patient health outcomes.

Alongside the problems of healthcare professionals' digital skills and awareness, another significant obstacle for the effective deployment of the new systems is posed by the multilevel governance in the Italian NHS. The digital transformation of Italy's National Health Service (NHS) has faced and still struggles with the significant challenges of its regional silos as a critical barrier to system-wide interoperability. The Italian NHS regional model has created profound disparities in the first adoption of the FSE, resulting in heterogeneous technological and organisational approaches across territories. This fragmentation has compromised both national interoperability and equitable access to digital health innovations for healthcare professionals, researchers, and patients.

The previous FSE regional implementation reveals a stark digital divide. High-performing regions like Emilia-Romagna and Lombardy have demonstrated successful FSE integration through (a) sustained investment in modern IT infrastructure; (b) adoption of HL7 FHIR interoperability standards; and (c) comprehensive clinician training programs. In contrast, lagging regions show persistent gaps, where (a) not all healthcare facilities regularly contribute to FSE data repositories; (b) most submitted data remains unstructured (PDFs, free-text); (c) IT legacy systems account for most of the local healthcare IT infrastructure.

This disparity has created a "two-tier" digital health ecosystem that undermines the FSE's potential for health data management and prevents its effective usage for nationwide policy making and research. The absence of standardised data collection protocols, clinical coding practices, and HIS interoperability frameworks has resulted in incomplete, inconsistent datasets unsuitable for advanced analytics or nationwide care coordination.

To address critical infrastructural barriers in regionally managed healthcare information systems, the new FSE 2.0 proposes a federated network with unified standards, which can, if well-coordinated in its implementation, significantly reduce regional disparities.

Another critical factor for the full deployment of FSE 2.0 and EDS potential is combining compliance with data protection rules and concerns with the need to make value of health data. The proposed governance framework for Italy's Health Data Ecosystem (EDS) also establishes a clear division of responsibilities, aligned with EU data protection principles. As mandated by Art. 4(7) GDPR, the Ministry of Health serves as the data controller, while the National Agency for Regional Health Services (Agenas) operates as a technical processor for infrastructure management (Ministry of Health, 2023).

The EDS will process Electronic Health Record (FSE 2.0) data for public interest purposes, including:

1. Synthetic health profile
2. Care process support
3. Pharmaceutical dossier
4. Health system monitoring, using OECD indicators for cross-national benchmarking

At the same time, it will ensure GDPR compliance through the implementation of:

- Art. 6(1)(e) for lawful processing
- Art. 25 for data minimisation protocols
- Art. 30 for activity logging

However, while the final implementation decrees are still in progress, there are still important points to be defined. Some technical specifications and requirements remain unclear, in terms of: (a) Anonymisation techniques (k-anonymity vs. differential privacy); (b) cross-border data sharing in the European Union; and (c) API standards (HL7 FHIR vs. openEHR).

Regulation (EU) 2025/327, establishing the European Health Data Space (EHDS), provides a timely framework for identifying final solutions, as it defines a set of standards, rules, and prescriptions that represent the first step towards the establishment of a "European Health Record" for every EU citizen. This should be a digital space in which all the clinical data defined as "priority" of each European citizen will be stored, including prescriptions, information on therapies, and the results of laboratory tests, even though each Member State will be entitled to add other "primary" categories. The relevance of EHDS lies not only in setting common standards for improved digitalisation of healthcare in Europe and in facilitating continuity of care across national borders, but also in being a strategic lever for the development of European health research based on real big data, with high ethical and scientific standards. Its implementation could be one of the main enablers for the predictive, personalised, and cooperative healthcare of the next decade.

7 Conclusions

The full implementation of the new Italian Electronic Health Record (FSE 2.0) and the Health Data Ecosystem (EDS) cannot be conceived as a simple infrastructure or regulatory compliance operation. On the contrary, it requires a strategic vision that transforms the project into a national pillar of digital health services, significantly transforming the status quo.

The EDS, as designed by the governmental guidelines, is conceived as an enabling and federable infrastructure, serving a more integrated and data-driven healthcare system. But for it to effectively fulfil this role, the system must be equipped with clear governance rules, shared responsibilities, and operational mechanisms, on top of the allocated investments in infrastructures and software.

The success of the ambitious new initiatives needs a comprehensive approach to overcome persistent fragmentation through synergistic interventions: (1) harmonised technical standardisation, (2) robust infrastructure development, (3) systematic capacity-building initiatives, and (4) clear new governance mechanisms between central government and Regions.

As highlighted in the European Health Data Space (EHDS) regulatory framework (European Parliament, 2024), to achieve nationwide interoperability, it is crucial to adopt open technical standards (HL7 FHIR R4+) within federated network architectures, coupled with active engagement of healthcare professionals across all levels of the healthcare system. However, the deployment of FSE 2.0/EDS represents more than a technological upgrade: it constitutes a fundamental transformation of Italy's digital health infrastructure. Drawing upon the digital health ecosystem framework, this initiative must evolve into a cornerstone of national health services, generating multidimensional value through clinical integration, operational efficiency, and research capacity.

The EDS functions as a federated infrastructure designed to support personalised, sustainable healthcare delivery. However, its effectiveness will need:

(a) Precisely defined governance protocols, delineating central-regional responsibilities
(b) Formalised interregional coordination structures, with binding service-level agreements
(c) Standardised interoperability metrics (e.g. API response times, data completeness)

The transition to a federated EDS model necessitates a fundamental reconfiguration of central-regional relations, shifting from vertical one-way flows to horizontal cooperation. The project's ultimate success will be determined not solely by technical specifications, but rather through the national system's capacity to implement mature innovative governance structures with continuous quality improvement cycles and regular monitoring.

Developing a federal model based on principles of reciprocal accountability in order to deploy the digital infrastructures needed for data-driven healthcare and health research will provide Italy with the opportunity to establish a renewed national healthcare system that will reduce regional disparities, overcome the digital divide, and result in a genuine "patient-centrism".

Bibliography

1. Arias JJ, Taylor J, O'Sullivan S (2022) Privacy and security in health data: challenges and opportunities in the era of digital health. J Med Internet Res 24(1):e34467
2. Casà C, Marotta C, Di Pumpo M, Cozzolino A, D'Aviero A, Frisicale EM, Silenzi A, Gabbrielli F, Bertinato L, Brusaferro S (2023) COVID-19 and digital competencies among young physicians: are we (really) ready for the new era? A national survey of the Italian Young Doctors Association. Ann Ist Super Sanita 57(1):1–6. https://annali.iss.it/index.php/anna/article/view/1170
3. Dash S, Shakyawar SK, Sharma M et al (2019) Big data in healthcare: management, analysis and future prospects. J Big Data 6:54. https://doi.org/10.1186/s40537-019-0217-0
4. Fanelli S, Pratici L, Salvatore F, Donelli C, Zangrandi A (2022) Big data analysis for decision making processes: challenges and opportunities for the management of health-care organizations. Manag Res Rev. issn:2040-8269
5. Marino A, Pariso P, Landriani L (2024) E-Health and Electronic Health Record: the Italian experience in the European context. https://doi.org/10.21203/rs.3.rs-31655/v1
6. Perrella A, Bisogno M (2025) The strength and resilience of Italy's health data system. Lancet Reg Health Eur 51:101255. https://doi.org/10.1016/j.lanepe.2025.101255. PMID: 40104393; PMCID: PMC11914812
7. Piscitelli P, Miani A, Schittulli F, Anelli F, Gesualdo L, Colao A (2025) Recognizing the limits of the 21 different Italian healthcare regional systems: an opportunity for change? Lancet Reg Health Eur 51:101250. https://doi.org/10.1016/j.lanepe.2025.101250. PMID: 40236448; PMCID: PMC11997440

8. Posteraro N, Corso S (2023) The Italian electronic health record (EHR). Eur Rev Digit Admin Law 4:187–200
9. Somayeh A, Hanke S, Hussein R (2025) Application of the openEHR reference model for PGHD: a case study on the DH-convener initiative. Int J Med Inform 193. https://doi.org/10.1016/j.ijmedinf.2024.105686. issn:1386-5056
10. Zarour M et al (2021) Ensuring data integrity of healthcare information in the era of digital health. Health Technol Lett 8:66–77. https://doi.org/10.1049/htl2.12008
11. Alessandra, Poggiani Agostino, Cortesi Khalid, Saeed Jiří, Dvorský (2024) Computer Information Systems and Industrial Management 23rd International Conference CISIM 2024 Bialystok Poland September 27–29 2024 Proceedings Challenges in Health Information Systems: Health Data Management and Access for Life Sciences Research Springer Nature Switzerland Cham 195-211
12. David, Natali Emmanuele, Pavolini Andrea, Terlizzi (2023) Multi-Level Governance Feedback and Health Care in Italy in the Aftermath of Covid-19 Politics and Governance 11(4) https://doi.org/10.17645/pag.i374 10.17645/pag.v11i4.7356
13. Tugce, Schmitt Shona, Cosgrove Vanja, Pajić Kimon, Papadopoulos Felix, Gille (2023) What does it take to create a European Health Data Space? International commitments and national realities Zeitschrift für Evidenz Fortbildung und Qualität im Gesundheitswesen 1791-7 https://doi.org/10.1016/j.zefq.2023.03.011
14. Muhammad, Ayaz Muhammad Fermi, Pasha Tahani Jaser, Alahmadi Nik Nailah Binti, Abdullah Hend Khalid, Alkahtani (2023) Transforming Healthcare Analytics with FHIR: A Framework for Standardizing and Analyzing Clinical Data Healthcare 11(12) 1729-10.3390/healthcare11121729

Chapter 7
A Comparison Between Health Data Sharing Normative Models

Beniamino Parenzo

1 Introduction and Overview

Health data indeed constitute a "special category" of personal data, not only in light of the fact that this is the formal qualification that they are given under Art. 9(1) of Reg. (EU) 2016/679 (so-called GDPR), but also by virtue of the actual and peculiar "intrinsic tension" they embody (to a greater extent than other "special categories" of personal data) between the data subject's need for their "seclusion" and the "openness" demands carried by the broader community.

While it is self-evident that the individuals to whom health data refer have a strong interest in keeping the "sensitive" information they reveal confidential, it is equally clear and undeniable that society has a vested interest in the broadest possible use (and reuse) of such data for a wide range of public purposes of "social utility", for which these data may prove instrumental. For instance, they may be of significant value for public health surveillance or for ensuring high levels of quality and safety in healthcare (see Art. 53(1)(a), Reg. (EU) 2025/327 on the European Health Data Space). They might serve policymaking and regulatory activities to support public sector bodies (see Art. 53(1)(b), Reg. (EU) 2025/327). Furthermore, their secondary processing could be used to improve the delivery of care, optimise treatment, and enhance the provision of healthcare (see Art. 53(1)(f), Reg. (EU) 2025/327), as well as, more generally, to foster scientific research in the healthcare sector (see Art. 53(1)(e) Reg. (EU) 2025/327).

Among the fundamental regulatory sources entrusted with balancing these (potentially) conflicting needs for "seclusion" and "openness", we first and foremost find Regulation (EU) 2016/679 (GDPR), which, as early as Recital (4), sets

B. Parenzo (✉)
Ca' Foscari University of Venice, Venice, Italy
e-mail: beniamino.parenzo@unive.it

A. Bernes, S. Thobani (eds.), *Digitalisation in Health Care between New Technologies, Data and Research*, Services and Business Process Reengineering, https://doi.org/10.1007/978-981-95-6982-3_7

out the methodological rule by which such conflict is to be resolved, stating: "The processing of personal data should be designed to serve mankind. The right to the protection of personal data is *not an absolute right*; it must be considered in relation to its *function in society* and be *balanced* against other fundamental rights, *in accordance with the principle of proportionality*". From this, the structure of the aforementioned Art. 9 of the GDPR becomes clear. After setting out, in paragraph 1, a categorical prohibition on the processing of special categories of personal data (including, notably, health data), it then opens, in paragraph 2, to the possibility of their use upon the occurrence of a series of (quite numerous, albeit stringent) exceptions.

However, it is not the regulatory framework established by the GDPR that will be addressed in the following discussion. Rather, by focusing on that specific type of processing which consists of the *sharing* of health data, the aim of this contribution is to analytically examine the different regulatory models of data sharing introduced by other, more recent acts adopted by the European legislator within the context of the so-called European Strategy for Data. More specifically, reference is made to Reg. (EU) 2022/868 on European data governance ("Data Governance Act"; hereinafter, "DGA") and to the already briefly mentioned Reg. (EU) 2025/327 on the European Health Data Space (hereinafter, "EHDS Regulation").

The purpose of the comparative analysis to be conducted is, more precisely, to assess how the different models of data sharing envisaged by these acts articulate the aforementioned balancing between the data subject's right to protection and the interests of third parties and of society at large, within a regulatory framework which is, quite evidently, programmatically geared toward an "opening" of health data to external use.

The analysis will begin with the two models introduced by the DGA, which are of a more strictly "private law" nature (considering that, in both cases, the sharing of health data is based on the data subject's consent). More specifically, after highlighting the fundamental shift introduced by the DGA with regard to data sharing—a shift away from the (more "static") protection-oriented perspective of the GDPR (Sect. 2)— the so-called data altruism provided for in Artt. 16 et seq. of the DGA will be examined (Sect. 3), followed by the analysis of that particular data intermediation service referred to in Art. 10(c) DGA, namely data cooperatives (Sect. 4). In this second model, it will be observed, the data subject's needs for protection and control are more thoroughly addressed than in the first one, where the balance tends, on the contrary, to tip more clearly in favour of the other pole.

This will be followed (Sect. 5) by an assessment of the predominantly public law-based framework set out by the EHDS Regulation concerning the secondary use of data. As will be noted, in this case the model adopted by the European legislator is clearly "tilted" toward promoting the reuse of health data: emblematic in this regard is the fact that secondary use can take place entirely *without the data subject's consent*, who is merely granted a "right to opt out".

2 From the GDPR to the DGA: From the Protection to the Sharing of Personal Data

In the EU regulatory landscape governing the so-called digital economy, the Data Governance Act marks a clear paradigm shift from the GDPR. More precisely, this shift can be concisely described as a transition from a system of *protection* to a regulatory framework for the *sharing* of personal data.

Indeed, even within the GDPR system itself, it is well known that the perspective was never one of an "absolutist" protection of personal data, understood as a "possession" of the individual to be "shielded" and "sheltered" from any form of external interference (an emblematic example in this regard is Recital (4) of the GDPR, already mentioned above). On the contrary, from the GDPR—and even earlier, from Directive 95/46/EC—the protection of personal data has never been aimed at securing a sort of isolation within the data subject's personal sphere. Rather, it is intended to be reconciled with, and balanced against, the demands of a digital market that, on the other hand, requires the free flow of such data.

Faced with such demands, the need for protection manifests not as a prohibition of circulation, but as a guarantee for the data subject to *exercise control* over that circulation. In this regulatory framework, protection and circulation of personal data operate in a reciprocal relationship, built around a general principle whereby the former does not negate the latter, but rather *shapes* it.

If it is therefore undoubtedly true that the framework established by the GDPR is built upon an axiological foundation where the guarantee of «a high level of protection of personal data» is considered a value co-essential to the need to «further facilitate the free flow of personal data» (see Recital (6) GDPR), then the framework introduced by the DGA represents such an "accelerated evolution" of that approach that it can be described in terms of a true paradigm shift: from a model in which protection gives shape to circulation, the focus of the European legislator now shifts toward the definition of a governance framework for the reuse and sharing of personal data.

While the need to protect data is by no means denied, the objective becomes that of establishing a regulatory framework aimed at further encouraging its circulation.

Whereas the GDPR focuses on the relationship between the data controller and the data subject—the former holding a qualified interest in processing the personal data of the latter, and the latter being protected in their interest to exercise control over such processing—the DGA moves beyond the boundaries of this "bilateral relationship" and broadens the regulatory perspective to encompass the further circulation of data. While the GDPR regulates the obligations that shape the data processing activities of the controller and the rights held by the data subject in relation to the controller, the DGA transcends this "individual space"—the space defined by the relationship between the principal actors of data processing—and instead shifts its normative focus toward the (new) actors involved in the reuse and sharing of personal data.

Furthermore, while under the GDPR, the perspective is essentially that of the "data subject–data controller" relationship, the DGA introduces a "*trilateral relationship*", involving a third party whose role is precisely to facilitate the further circulation of data.

The normative model established by the DGA can be summarised as follows: a party (who does not necessarily coincide with the "data subject", but may also be a "data holder", defined in Art. 2(8) DGA as "a legal person [...] or a natural person who is not a data subject with respect to the specific data in question, which [...] has the right to grant access to or to share certain personal data") shares data with third parties (the so-called data users—see Art. 2(9) DGA), through the intermediation of a designated "data intermediary".

If, as previously noted, under the DGA the sharing of data occurs exclusively on a voluntary basis—that is, upon the initiative and consent of the party entitled to make such data available—then, depending on the "nature" of the intermediary and the purposes pursued through its mediation service, two distinct models of data sharing can be identified, which essentially differ in that the data sharing service is carried out for profit or for solidarity purposes. In the former case, data sharing is carried out through "data intermediation services" (Artt. 10 et seq. DGA); in the latter, through "data altruism organisations" (Artt. 16 et seq. DGA).

As previously mentioned, the following sections will take a closer look at these two models—data altruism and data intermediation services (in particular, in the form of data cooperatives)—with the aim of highlighting how the former tends to promote the kind of "socially functional" openness previously discussed, while the latter is more explicitly oriented toward strengthening and empowering the position of the data subject.

3 Data Altruism

Data altruism is defined by Art. 2(16) DGA as "the voluntary sharing of data on the basis of the consent of data subjects to process personal data pertaining to them [...] without seeking or receiving a reward that goes beyond compensation related to the costs that they incur where they make their data available for objectives of general interest as provided for in national law, where applicable, such as healthcare, combating climate change, improving mobility, facilitating the development, production and dissemination of official statistics, improving the provision of public services, public policy making or scientific research purposes in the general interest".

According to its definition, this model would indeed appear to represent the "natural" or "inherent" mode of sharing health data: a form of solidaristic "donation" of sensitive data aimed at contributing to the achievement of objectives of general interest, such as, among others, healthcare and scientific research.

In its essential provisions, the detailed regulation ultimately rests on a series of measures which, precisely due to the "social utility" performed by this (private) instrument of data sharing, aim to ensure (public-law style) oversight over the entities through which such activity is carried out, as well as over the data sharing activity itself.

More specifically, the following "key points" can be identified:

1. Entities intending to carry out data altruism activities are subject to a registration requirement with a public national register of recognised data altruism organisations (see Artt. 17 et seq. DGA), conditional upon verification of the requirements set forth in Art. 18 DGA (among which it is required that the organisation in question be a not-for-profit legal person)
2. The activity carried out must comply with a series of transparency obligations, concretised in the maintenance of registers and the submission of an annual report to the competent authority on the activities performed (see Art. 20 DGA), as well as specific obligations towards the data subjects (see Art. 21 DGA), which will be examined in more detail shortly
3. The competent authorities responsible for the registration of data altruism organisations are vested with the power to monitor and supervise compliance of data altruism organisations with the provisions established by the Regulation, as well as the power to sanction any violations found (see Art. 24 DGA).

The circulatory model in question, as briefly anticipated above, is more "tilted" towards promoting greater data sharing rather than strict control by the data subject, with a resulting heightened "focus" on third-party users rather than on the data subject themselves (which, however, is by no means inconsistent, but rather aligned with the *solidaristic* nature of the sharing itself).

This is clearly evidenced by the provision set forth in Art. 21 DGA. First and foremost, it is indeed indicative that the provision stipulates that a data altruism organisation "*shall provide tools for obtaining consent from data subjects*" (Art. 21(3) DGA); indeed, from the perspective of the data user, the data altruism organisation acts as a "*less than neutral*" intermediary, with its activity aimed, among other things, at «*facilitating* data processing by third parties». Accordingly, it must endeavour to provide these parties with the "tools" necessary to obtain the consent of the data subjects (see Art. 21(6) DGA).

Equally emblematic, secondly, is the fact that while Art. 21(3) DGA establishes the obligation for the data altruism organisation to provide tools for the easy withdrawal of consent, nothing else is stipulated in this regard: in particular, there is no mention of the exercise of rights granted to the data subject under the GDPR, and thus, for example, no obligation on the part of the data altruism organisation to provide tools to facilitate the exercise of those rights (unlike what is established for data intermediation services, as we will see shortly in the next paragraph).

Thirdly and finally, consideration must be given to the provision set forth in Art. 21(1)(a) DGA, which is not only indicative with respect to the discussion we are conducting but also rather problematic when compared to the protective provisions established by the GDPR. This provision places an obligation on the data altruism organisation to "inform data subjects or data holders prior to any processing of their data in a clear and easily comprehensible manner of [...] the objectives of general interest and, if applicable, the specified, explicit and legitimate purpose for which personal data is to be processed, and for which it permits the processing of their data by a data user".

The information obligation established appears, in its minimal content, to be limited solely to the "objectives of general interest" for which the data are shared, potentially concerning the specific purposes of processing only "*if appropriate*". Provocatively, one could argue that insofar as the specific purposes of processing may not be disclosed to the data subject, the solidaristic sharing that takes place within the framework of data altruism could ultimately amount to a kind of "blanket delegation" for processing. As noted, this is rather problematic, as such a provision is clearly at odds with the so-called principle of purpose limitation set forth in Art. 5(1)(b) GDPR, which explicitly requires that the data subject be accurately informed of the *explicit and specific purposes* of the processing.

With regard to the contradiction now identified, one could certainly argue that, on closer inspection, the GDPR also sets out a derogation from the principle of purpose limitation, insofar as Recital 33 of the GDPR seems to admit the possibility of "broad consent" for processing for scientific research purposes. Considered that "it is often not possible to fully identify the purpose of personal data processing for scientific research purposes at the time of data collection" it is given the possibility that data subjects might "give their consent to *certain areas* of scientific research". In this regard, however, it is worth mentioning the opinion expressed by the European Data Protection Board ("EDPB") in its Guidelines 05/2020 on consent under Regulation 2016/679, which after having found that "Recital 33 seems to bring some flexibility to the degree of specification and granularity of consent in the context of scientific research", nonetheless states that "Recital 33 does not disapply the obligations with regard to the requirement of specific consent". Consequently, two options are identified in order to balance the principle of specific consent with the impossibility to fully specify at the outset of the research its specific purposes: (1) either that of a "progressive consent", which requires that as the research advances, consent for subsequent steps in the project shall be obtained before that next stage begins; (2) or that of a "progressive disclosure" obligation, according to which "a lack of purpose specification may be offset by information on the development of the purpose being provided regularly by controllers as the research project progresses so that, over time, the consent will be as specific as possible". These same solutions should also be considered applicable with respect to the consent given by the data subject for the sharing of their data in the context of data altruism, as provided by the DGA.

4 Data Intermediation Services: Data Cooperatives

The model established by the regulation on intermediation services—and in particular on data cooperatives—appears to be quite different.

Art. 2(11) DGA defines a "data intermediation service" as a "service which aims to establish commercial relationships for the purposes of data sharing between an undetermined number of data subjects and data holders on the one hand and data users on the other". The Regulation then identifies in Art. 10 three types of intermediation services: "(a) intermediation services between data holders and potential data users [...]; (b) intermediation services between data subjects that seek to make their personal data available or natural persons that seek to make non-personal data available, and potential data users, including making available the technical or other means to enable such services, and in particular enabling the exercise of the data subjects' rights provided in Regulation (EU) 2016/679; (c) services of data cooperatives". As previously mentioned, particular attention will be given to the third type.

Indeed, while it is certainly true that, in general, all intermediation services offering services to data subjects are expressly required to act "in the data subjects' *best interest* where it facilitates the exercise of their rights, in particular by informing and, where appropriate, advising data subjects in a concise, transparent, intelligible and easily accessible manner about intended data uses by data users and standard terms and conditions attached to such uses before data subjects give consent" (see Art. 12(m) DGA); with specific regard to data cooperatives, these appear to be, "by their very nature", the type of service that best embodies, through their participatory structure, the pursuit of that "best interest" of the data subjects.

As can be inferred from the definition provided in Art. 2(15) of the DGA: (1) data cooperatives constitute "organisational structures" (not further defined in terms of their legal nature—deliberately so, it must be assumed, in order to allow for greater flexibility in application of the concept), of which the data subjects themselves are members; (2) "having as its main objectives to support its members in the exercise of their rights with respect to certain data, including with regard to making informed choices before they consent to data processing, to exchange views on data processing purposes and conditions that would best represent the interests of its members in relation to their data, and to negotiate terms and conditions for data processing on behalf of its members [...] before they consent to the processing of personal data".

In other words, this is a decidedly *sui generis* intermediation service compared to the other two types of services provided for under Art. 10 of the DGA. It is a service that is by no means "neutral" in its very foundational structure and is, in fact, institutionally "partial". Its corporate purpose is precisely—as is typical of any "associative organisation" (to use a formula as generic as the one employed by the European legislator) with a mutualistic aim—to assist its members in making informed and conscious decisions regarding the circulation of their personal data and (in cases of data circulation for remuneration) in negotiating better contractual terms with third parties. It must also certainly be considered possible for the data subject to delegate to the data cooperative the exercise of the rights granted by the GDPR.

Without any rhetorical overstatement, one may therefore resort to a somewhat predictable—yet in this case undeniably fitting—slogan: in a data cooperative, "unity is strength".

In other words, and to put it differently, in the case of data altruism, the data subject's condition is not, in truth, substantially different from the "standard" condition assigned to them by the GDPR. That is, while they are formally granted a set of rights intended to ensure their control over the circulation of their data, the actual effectiveness of this control risks being undermined in practice by the difficulties they may encounter in exercising those rights.

By contrast, in the case of a data cooperative, it is precisely the fact that the circulation and subsequent control of the data occur through a "collective structure" which helps the data subject to understand the purposes and conditions of the processing, and which—*acting in their best interest*—negotiates with third parties the terms of the processing and exercises, on their behalf, the rights that ensure such control. In this way, the data subject is placed in a real position to be an informed and active participant in the processes involving the circulation of their data.

In summary, whereas under the GDPR system—which undoubtedly applies to the circulatory mechanisms of data altruism—the data subject is ultimately "alone", both at the moment of giving consent to data processing and later when seeking to exercise the rights that are meant to ensure control over the circulation of their data, in the cooperative system, they find renewed strength precisely through the collective structure. It is through this structure that they are able to become an effective interlocutor in circulatory processes that would otherwise remain opaque and "alien" to them.

All of this, of course, without ever losing the ability to make individual decisions regarding data processing or to exercise their rights on an individual basis (indeed, the collective dimension never amounts to a denial or "overriding" of the individual one, but rather serves as its "amplification", its "empowerment").

In conclusion, with regard to the two private law models governed by the DGA, while it is true that, at first glance, data altruism might appear to be the "natural" or "physiological" model within which to frame the circulation of that particular category of data constituted by health data, a more in-depth analysis reveals that, precisely in light of the close connection of such data to the individual and their particularly heightened "sensitivity", the participatory model represented by the data cooperative can, if one seeks to prioritise the need for stronger protection of the data subject, undoubtedly be considered the preferable option.

5 Secondary Use of Health Data Under the EHDS Regulation

Among the other objectives pursued, Reg. (EU) 2025/327 establishing the European Health Data Space(hereinafter "EHDS") lays down common rules and mechanisms for secondary use of electronic health data (see Art. 1(2)(c)), i.e. "for processing of data for purposes other than those for which they were collected or produced" (see Recital 55). The aim is to overcome the fragmentation that has so far characterised the further circulation of health data, which has been regulated differently across Member States, and instead to establish a common framework intended to facilitate and promote the circulation of health data in order to fully unleash their potential "in the general interest of society" (see Recital 61).

The Regulation establishes a public system for access to electronic health data, governed through the intermediation of the so-called Health Data Access Bodies.

In a nutshell, the envisaged sharing model is the following: a person or entity intending to use health data for one of the permitted secondary use purposes (a "health data user") may submit an application for access to data to the Health Data Access Body. The requested data must fall into one or more of the categories of electronic health data listed in Art. 51 and must be held by a "health data holder" (defined in Art. 2(2)(t) as "any natural or legal person, public authority, agency or other body in the healthcare or care sectors"). The application must specify the intended purposes and characteristics of the proposed processing (see Art. 67). Upon receipt of the application, the Health Data Access Body decides whether to issue a "data permit"—that is, an *administrative decision* authorising the processing of the specified electronic health data for the indicated secondary use purposes (see Art. 2(2)(v)).

As is evident, this is a mechanism entirely *detached from the need for the data subject's consent*, who is, ultimately, not involved at any stage of the procedure. The only power granted to the data subject, a sort of "negative control", consists in a «right to opt out at any time, and without providing any reason, from the processing of personal electronic health data» (see Art. 71).

The intention guiding and supporting the regulatory framework established by the EHDS Regulation for the secondary use of health data is, in essence, clearly aimed at promoting the need for *openness* of health data in order to more effectively pursue the interests of the broader community.

Particularly indicative in this regard are the exhaustive list of purposes under Art. 53 for which secondary use is permitted, namely purposes: (a) in the public interest in the field of public health or occupational medicine; (b) supporting public entities in policy making activities in the healthcare or care sectors; (c) compiling statistics related to the healthcare or care sectors; (d) education or teaching in the healthcare or care sectors; (e) scientific research in the healthcare or care sectors; (f) improving and optimising the delivery of care services.

Equally emblematic is the obligation laid down in Art. 61(4) requiring data users to make public «the results or output of secondary use, including information relevant for the provision of healthcare, within 18 months of the completion of the processing of the electronic health data»; as well as the obligations imposed on Health Data Access Bodies under Art. 58, according to which, they "shall make information on the conditions under which electronic health data are made available for secondary use publicly available, easily searchable through electronic means and accessible for natural persons", information which, among the others, shall cover "who has been granted access to datasets of electronic health data and to which datasets they were granted access and details of the data permit regarding the purposes for processing such data" (Art. 53(1)(f)) and "the results or outcomes of the projects for which the electronic health data were used" (Art. 53(1)(g)).

Although the model established by the European legislator is clearly "tilted" in favour of the reuse of health data in the public interest, it must nevertheless be emphasised that this does not, conversely, entail a sacrifice of the need to protect individuals.

First and foremost, the axiological centrality of the GDPR remains firmly upheld: compliance with the GDPR must, in any case, be demonstrated by the data user in order to obtain a data permit (see Art. 68(1)(c)) for the secondary use of health data: "When seeking access to the personal electronic health data in a pseudonymised format—enshrines Art. 67(4)—the health data applicant shall provide, together with the health data access application, a description of how the processing would comply with [...] Regulation (EU) 2016/679 and, more specifically, with Art. 6(1) thereof".

Highly significant, among others, are also the provisions set forth in Artt. 66 and 73. Art. 66 reiterates the well-known principles of data minimisation and purpose limitation (see Art. 5 GDPR): "Where health data access bodies receive a health data access application, they shall ensure that access is only provided to electronic health data that are adequate, relevant and limited to what is necessary in relation to the purpose of processing indicated in the health data access application". Furthermore, following a hierarchy of preferences already established by Art. 89 GDPR, it is also provided that health data access bodies shall provide anonymised data, and only where the health data user has sufficiently demonstrated that the purpose of processing cannot be achieved, they shall provide access to electronic health data in a pseudonymised format (keeping secret, however, the information necessary to reverse the pseudonymization).

The second provision, on the other hand, provides that "health data access bodies shall provide access to electronic health data pursuant to a data permit *only through a secure processing environment* which is subject to technical and organisational measures and security and interoperability requirements" and that they "shall review the electronic health data included in a download request to ensure that health data users are only able to download non-personal electronic health data". In other terms, secondary circulation does not involve any transfer of personal data from the data holder to the data user; the latter, upon obtaining the data permit, is solely authorised to access and process such data within the secure processing environment provided by the Health Data Access Body, without the possibility of downloading them except in anonymised form.

In overall conclusion, while the new framework established by the European legislator certainly does not abandon the system of protections guaranteed by the GDPR (whose axiological centrality remains unquestioned), what appears to have significantly changed in this new context of secondary circulation of health data is precisely the model of data circulation itself. Alongside the "publicization" of the purposes of circulation, the governance and control system also sees the "private" role of data subjects and data processors notably diminish, being instead assigned to these new administrative authorities—the Health Data Access Bodies—called upon to play a decisive role both in the circulation of data and in the implementation of protective measures.

Bibliography

1. Bravo F (2023) Le cooperative di dati. Contratto e impresa 3:757–799
2. Bravo F (ed) (2024) EU Data Cooperatives. L'ingresso delle cooperative di dati nell'ordinamento europeo. Giappichelli, Torino
3. Morace PA (2024) Dalla data protection alla data governance: il Regolamento UE 2022/868. Nuova giurisprudenza civile commentata 2:486–495
4. Nuccio MR (2023) Digitalizzazione e circolazione dei dati sanitari. Tecnologie e diritto 2:357–376
5. Owusu A (2022) Data sharing in the personal data economy. Does sharing mean caring? Eur J Privacy Law Technol 2:217–239
6. Perlingieri C, Cocco A (2024) 'Primary' and 'secondary' use of electronic health data. Ital Law J 10:275–295
7. Poletti D (2022) Gli intermediari dei dati. Eur J Privacy Law Technol 1:45–56
8. Quinn P, Ellyne E, Yao C (2024) Will the GDPR restrain health data access bodies under the European Health Data Space (EHDS)? Comput Law Secur Rev 54:1–15
9. Rapisarda I (2021) Ricerca scientifica e circolazione dei dati personali. Verso il definitivo superamento del paradigma privatistico? Eur Dirit Priv 2:301–347
10. Terzis P (2023) Compromises and asymmetries in the European Health Data Space. Eur J Health Law 30:345–363
11. Terzis P, Santamaria Echeverria OE (2023) Interoperability and governance in the European Health Data Space regulation. Med Law Int 23:368–376

Part II
Technologies, Artificial Intelligence and Liability

Chapter 8
Technological Innovation and Medical Robots

Giovanni Di Rosa

1 State of the Art and Plan of the Investigation

The Italian health care context is today affected by profound transformations to which certain reforms attempt to provide appropriate responses. These reforms, attempting to take stock of what has unfortunately happened due to the recent pandemic emergency, aim to ensure the best conditions for health protection, within an overall reorganization of the socio-health care system. Moreover, it cannot be overlooked that, at this precise moment in history, the generally invoked principle of health care sustainability, i.e., the ability to provide high-quality health care today without compromising the ability of future generations to provide equally good health care in turn, must come to terms with the principle of demographic sustainability. In fact, our country is, after Japan, the oldest in the world, counting as many as 14 million retirees and seven million children, with 24% of the population over the age of 65, and, conversely, has one of the lowest fertility rates in the world, at 1.2 children per woman, with one of the highest life expectancies, namely 84 years.

It is, therefore, inevitable to question whether it is really possible to ensure health care rights, while also guaranteeing the maintenance of certain quality standards. In this regard, Law No. 33 of March 23, 2023, delegating to the government policies in favor of the elderly person, and Legislative Decree No. 29 of March 15, 2024, containing provisions on policies in favor of the elderly person, can be pointed out. The aforementioned measures aim in good substance, both in general terms, that is,

The paper is a product of the UNICT University Research Program 2020–2022, line 2, "New assets, technological innovation and protection techniques."

G. Di Rosa (✉)
University of Catania, Catania, Italy
e-mail: gdirosa@lex.unict.it

A. Bernes, S. Thobani (eds.), *Digitalisation in Health Care between New Technologies, Data and Research*, Services and Business Process Reengineering, https://doi.org/10.1007/978-981-95-6982-3_8

as far as policy criteria are concerned, and in particular terms, that is, as far as the corresponding implementation is concerned, to prevent the institutionalization of non-self-sufficient elderly persons, to strengthen (by integrating them) home-based services and telemedicine, and to strengthen intermediate health care and related facilities, in a context of increasing professionalization and empowerment of all those involved.

The central issue today, therefore, is the quality and accessibility of health care services, in an overall framework in which the so-called universalistic system, that is, the guarantee for all those who reside in the country of access to health care, regardless of their economic or social status, as ensured through public financing, is actually something different. Indeed, we are in the presence of a system with respect to which, in view of the scarcity of available resources, the least expensive services are in fact paid for by citizens.

In the face of the noted criticalities, both with regard to the factors that negatively affect (aging of the population, demographic winter, increase in chronic diseases) and with regard to the not entirely appropriate way of dealing with them (as it is believed to have happened in terms of a real application deficit as to the same recent reform of the social-health system), one of the possible, and by many parties highlighted, levers for making a significant turnaround is technological innovation (telemedicine, health data management systems, artificial intelligence applications) in order to optimize care processes and reduce related costs.

As for, in particular, artificial intelligence or robotic algorithmic systems, it is possible here to sketch their relative characters with respect to their possible legal implications. On the one hand, therefore, some possible typologies of them will be identified; on the other hand, correlatively, a corresponding, naturally diverse, legal configuration will be outlined. No less relevant, however, are the ethical issues and the correlative orders of problems that the aforementioned algorithmic applications in health care may determine. It may be briefly noted here, by way of a very brief mention, the necessary and permanent centrality of the doctor-patient relationship, because of the peculiar relationship between the activity required of the former and the type of care in favor of the latter.

2 Health Care Activities and Robotic Systems. Application Models and Functional Destinations

The identification, so to speak, typological of robotic applications in medicine is certainly preliminary in order to be able, precisely by moving to the technical configuration, i.e., what it is about from the technological point of view, then to turn to the correlative legal configuration, i.e., what are the legal aspects that come into consideration in order to be able to prepare the relevant regulation, whether adaptive or innovative.

As for the first profile (technical configuration), the already proposed distinction between two levels can be taken up here: one of a general character, and the other of a particular character. With regard to the distinction of a general character, thus independent of the relative scope of use, it is possible to recall the distinction between tele-operated robots, autonomous robots, and cognitive robots, that is, because of the different ways of acting in the human–machine relationship. In this regard, noting the absence of an unambiguous definition of robots on the technological side, the nonetheless obvious diversity from humans is expressed by pointing out that robots have remained, at least for the time being, artificial agents that perform tasks in place of humans and do so (more or less) autonomously.

Thus, we range from the simple mechanical instrument in the hands of an operator, who decides what actions to take, moreover performed under his close and constant control, to systems of maximum autonomy, for this reason considered "intelligent," capable not only of having their own representation of the external context of operation, but also of significant adaptability to the changing nature of the environment that surrounds them and with which they interact, that is, denoting the particular cognitive character and differing, for this reason, from systems of lesser and more limited autonomy.

With regard, on the other hand, to the health sector, it is stressed, on the one hand, a progressive development of the market with respect to the production activity and the corresponding release of (more or less) developed systems based on artificial intelligence. At the same time, however, on the other hand, the risk is pointed out that these same systems can sometimes generate illusory and misleading expectations, both for health professionals and for patients, apart from the new (but still ordinary) problems as to the related liability profiles, precisely in relation to any damage caused to the patients themselves.

With respect, then, to the correlative, punctual applications, it is possible to distinguish between clinical robotics, rehabilitative robotics, and assistive robotics, within which it is then possible to prospect a specific distinction because of the way through which, based on the type of machine used (more or less autonomous), the decision-making result is obtained with respect to the types of problems entrusted to the robotic solution.

With reference to clinical robotics, both clinico-medical and clinico-surgical systems can be reported, depending on their respective intended use for direct observation and study of the patient, and corresponding non-surgical therapeutic treatment (i.e., medical), or surgical therapeutic treatment (i.e., interventional).

The first group and the correlative typology include, for example, the Cyberknife robotic system, which is used in the field of so-called surgical radiotherapy (or radiosurgery). This denomination (apparently in contrast to the distinction previously envisaged) is due not so much to the realization of an actual surgical procedure (which it is not), but rather because a result similar (in terms of precision) to an actual surgical procedure (characterized by the surgical incision) is made possible through one or (normally) more sessions of radiotherapy treatment. Thus, it is a tool of advanced technology in the oncological arena, complementing the already established surgical, pharmacological, and radiotherapy practices, deputed to send a high dose of high-power ionizing radiation, centered very precisely on the tumor, lesions, or other areas to be treated with a (possibly) minimal effect (far less than with traditional radiotherapy) on the surrounding healthy tissues.

The second group and the related group include the Da Vinci Surgical System medical robot, the most advanced apparatus in the field of minimally invasive surgery. This is a robot that operates through remote commands from a surgeon who sits at the console, i.e., uses a control instrument to remotely manage the movements of the robotic system, thereby operating its related mechanical arms on which the operating instruments are mounted. Corresponding to the very high cost, not only in terms of purchase but also in terms of maintenance and, likewise, training of health care personnel, there are several advantages, particularly reduced invasiveness and increased precision.

For rehabilitation robotics, one may recall, among others, the Lokomat system, a robotic exoskeleton intended to ensure the recovery of lower limb function. It allows the patient, through a system of harnesses that hold him upright, to perform leg movements on a treadmill through the robotic limbs to which the lower limbs are attached, based on motor patterns corresponding to those of ordinary, natural locomotion. To this order of systems also belongs, albeit with a different rehabilitative goal, ICub, the humanoid robot used effectively, within a proper clinical protocol, in interactions with young patients with autism spectrum disorder, i.e., a heterogeneous set of neurodevelopmental disorders that begin during developmental age and are characterized by deficits in communication and social interaction.

Care robotics refers to all those automated tools, which are increasingly numerous, intended to carry out common nursing activities (with a significant reduction of workloads for the related personnel) but also directed, more generally, to ensure adequate services to the person. Precisely with respect to the latter sector and type of activity may recall the humanoid robot Pepper (translation of pepper, chilli pepper, referring, by translation, to liveliness and vitality), which presents traits of significant interactivity. It is, in fact, able to move in its surroundings (moving on its wheels), recognize a human face, and perceive (through special sensors) the emotions of the people with whom it enters into a relationship. In particular, in some health care facilities, such a robot has been intended, within pediatric wards, to support professional figures as a facilitator of the relationship between the figure of the doctor (or other health care professional) and young patients. It is, therefore, a tool deputed to improve the quality of care and reduce the discomfort of the stay of young patients in the inpatient facility.

3 Problematic Reflections and Regulatory Perspectives

As, finally, to the second profile (legal configuration), with respect to the different typology, as referred to above, of medical robotic systems, one can highlight problems related now to the different degree of incidence of the machine in the relationship with the patient and between the health care provider and the patient himself;

now to the greater or lesser effectiveness of the use of such tools with respect to the activity of man; now, finally, to the issues in terms of liability arising from their use, more or less dangerous.

Moreover, the very transition from the merely instrumental character of the robotic means to the quite different substantially decisional trait of the automated "intelligent" system determines a different consideration and evaluation of the above orders of problems. It is sufficient in this regard to draw attention to the obvious difference between, for example, an automated activity directed to the acquisition and storage of health data and that directed to the subsequent use of the same with therapeutic decision-making functions, in a path that therefore still winds (but certainly with undoubted differences) through robotic systems. Just as, in the same way, the different robotic typology implies, with respect to the relative legal framework for the purposes of corresponding liability, different degrees of risk, certainly greater for invasive devices for surgical use, or in contact with the central nervous system.

On the one hand, therefore, there are issues of efficiency, not only in quantitative terms but also in qualitative terms, with clear repercussions in ethical terms with respect to the related impact on the relationship with the patient; on the other hand, there are issues of liability with respect to which the regulatory challenge has just begun. In the latter regard, in fact, two important regulatory steps can be recalled, one (supranational) having reached an initial conclusion, and the other (in domestic law) in progress.

As for the former, the final drafting of the first AI Act, passed last March 13, 2024 and published in the form of the EU Regulation, June 13, 2024, No. 1689 (Artificial Intelligence Act, acronym AI Act) in the EU Official Journal, July 12, 2024, should be noted. The regulation entered into force 20 days after its publication (thus, on August 2, 2024) and is expected to be fully implemented in the following 24 months (thus, from August 2, 2026). Its adoption was then followed by the signing by the European Commission of the Council of Europe Framework Convention on Artificial Intelligence on behalf of the European Union, the first legally binding international agreement on the subject; it provides a common approach to ensure that artificial intelligence systems are compatible with human rights, democracy, and the rule of law while enabling innovation and trust. The regulation is the result of a series of acts, starting with the proposed EU regulation, April 21, 2021, and the subsequent proposal for a European directive, September 28, 2022, on the European approach to artificial intelligence, an expression of the first European legal framework in this area. It was then approved by the European Parliament, on June 14, 2023, the final and amended (in a more protective sense) version of the aforementioned proposal of April 21, 2021, on which a preliminary agreement was reached, on December 9, 2023, between the Council, Parliament, and the EU Commission, which was followed by the final drafting and approval of the aforementioned AI Act.

The overall objective of the introduced regulation is to ensure that artificial intelligence systems used in the European Union are safe, transparent, traceable, non-discriminatory, and environmentally friendly, promoting "the deployment of anthropocentric and reliable artificial intelligence, while ensuring a high level of protection of health, safety and fundamental rights as enshrined in the Charter of Fundamental Rights of the European Union" (Recital 1).

Moreover, our Council of Ministers, in its session of April 23, 2024, approved, with the provision of the request to the Chambers for prompt calendaring in respect of the two branches of Parliament, a bill for the introduction of provisions and delegation to the Government on artificial intelligence (communicated to the Presidency of the Senate of the Republic on May 20, 2024), without any overlap with what has been approved in the EU, but accompanied (in an anthropocentric view) by the regulatory framework in the spaces proper to domestic law, taking into account that (as will be better represented shortly) the EU regulation is set on an architecture of risks related to the use of artificial intelligence. This internal initiative was then followed in July 2024 by the drafting of the document on the Italian Artificial Intelligence Strategy 2024–2026, which was prepared by a committee of experts to support the Italian government in defining national legislation and policies on artificial intelligence. The European Commission, however, making use of the power granted to it by EU Directive 2015/1535, aimed at protecting the single European space also with respect to the implementation by member states of European rules in the field of technical regulations and information society services, sent the Italian government a critical opinion with respect to the draft law on artificial intelligence, currently under consideration by the Senate of the Republic.

For what may be of immediate interest here, and in relation to the typological distinctions outlined above, it should be noted that central to the European framework is precisely the role of risk and the related adoption of harmonized liability rules. It has thus introduced a common objective (or no-fault) liability regime for artificial intelligence (autonomous) systems, and a common subjective (or no-fault) liability regime for artificial intelligence (autonomous) systems. Through correlative different provisions for the different types of risks, a common regime of strict liability (or no-fault) applies to (autonomous) artificial intelligence systems with high inherent risk, while a regime of subjective liability (or fault) applies to all other artificial intelligence systems (therefore not autonomous and in the absence of high inherent risk). This solution is useful to put in close correlation, precisely, the distinct types of artificial intelligence systems, notably high risk and firm the prohibition as to unacceptable risk, and the corresponding modalities of entry into the circuit of use, with the related identification of the subjects who may have to do with them (albeit with different roles) with respect to the obligations incumbent on each (supplier, distributor, user), with the aim of ensuring adequate standards of protection and, above all, ensuring the predetermination of different levels of responsibility.

Bibliography

1. Amato S (2020) Biodiritto 4.0. Intelligenza artificiale e nuove tecnologie. Giappichelli, Torino
2. Datteri E (2010) Danni senza anomalie; questioni di responsabilità nella robotica medica. Informatica e diritto 6:59–77
3. Di Rosa G (2025) Robot e responsabilità sanitaria. In: Albanese A, Guffanti Pesenti L, Tommasi S (eds) Il diritto privato nell'economia digitale. Giappichelli, Torino, pp 217–231
4. Di Rosa G (2022) I robot medici, Persona e mercato, pp 12–19
5. Finocchiaro G (2024) Intelligenza artificiale. Quali regole? Il Mulino, Bologna
6. Iagnemma C (2020) I 'robot medici': profili problematici in tema di alleanza terapeutica e di responsabilità penale. Corti supreme e salute 2:1–18
7. Marchese A (2021) Profili civilistici dell'information technology in àmbito sanitario. Edizioni Scientifiche Italiane, Napoli
8. Palmerini E (2016) Robotica e diritto, Responsabilità civile e previdenza, pp 1816–1850
9. Rapisarda I (2021) Ricerca scientifica e circolazione dei dati personali. Verso il superamento del paradigma privatistico? Europa e diritto privato, pp 301–347
10. Santosuosso A, Boscarato C, Caroleo F (2012) Robotica e diritto: una prima ricognizione. Nuova giurisprudenza civile commentata Pt. 2:494–516

Chapter 9
Between Civil Liability and Risk Governance: AI as a Medical Device

Valentina Calderai

1 Introduction

'It is difficult to imagine a sharper contrast than that presented by the EU today: the most refined and sophisticated legal scholarship in the world, and a positive law that seems to have deliberately freed itself from it. This law is built on rough and approximate language structures consisting of a few essential and repeated elements. These elements are similar to suburban neighbourhoods crowded with public housing: all identical and bleak' [1].

Carlo Castronovo's caustic judgement aptly describes the European model of technological risk governance. Product safety regulation within the New Legislative Framework (NLF) is quintessentially modular and iterative. This approach is based on the division of labour between traditional institutional sources and technical standards Here, the Commission firmly controls the levers of the machine, supported by expert committees. These committees play a crucial role as *relais* between public regulators and private standardisation organisations (European Standard Organisations: ESO): The European Committee for Standardisation (CEN), the European Committee for Electrotechnical Standardisation (CENELEC), and the European Telecommunications Standards Institute (ETSI).

The tension between classical law and regulation is particularly evident in the field of artificial intelligence-based medical devices (AI-MDs). This paper analyses how safety regulation in this sector has become the determining factor in the trade-off between innovation and safety, with significant implications for liability rules. The article proceeds as follows: the first section examines the architecture of the NLF and the ambiguous role of standardisation harmonisation; the second section

V. Calderai (✉)
University of Pisa, Pisa, Italy
e-mail: valentina.calderai@unipi.it

A. Bernes, S. Thobani (eds.), *Digitalisation in Health Care between New Technologies, Data and Research*, Services and Business Process Reengineering, https://doi.org/10.1007/978-981-95-6982-3_9

analyses the specific case of AI-MDs within the framework of Regulation (EU) No 1689/2024 on artificial intelligence (hereafter referred to as the 'AI Act'); the third section explores the relationship between safety and liability rules; and the final section identifies three trends and proposes reforms to increase the accountability of standardisation bodies.

2 The Architecture of the New Legislative Framework

2.1 From Voluntary Standards to Union Rules

The NLF is not actually new. The original framework dates back to the early 1980s. In a climate marked by a powerful drive towards economic globalisation, the WTO published the first version of the 'Principles for the Development of International Standards, Guides and Recommendations' (Six Principles), the most notable of which was consensus: 'Consensus procedures should be established that seek to take into account the views of all parties concerned and to reconcile any conflicting arguments'(see the WTO Agreement on Technical Barriers to Trade and the WTO-TBT Committee's Decision on Principles for the Development of International Standards, Guides and Recommendations in relation to Art. 2, 5 and Annex 3 of the WTO Agreement).

Consensus is linked to the definition of a technical standard as a document 'approved by a recognised body that provides rules, guidelines or characteristics for products or related processes and production methods, with which compliance is not mandatory' (WTO Agreement on Technical Barriers to Trade, Annex 1, Terms and Definitions).

From inception to enforcement, everything about standards seems to refer to a consensual and non-coercive dimension of private ordering, in tacit but sharp contrast with the vertical and centralised regulation of public institutions: 'a way of circumventing the arduous and cumbersome process of political decision-making' [2].

2.2 The Harmonised Standardisation Procedure

The formal integration of standardisation into the regulatory architecture of the European Economic Communities dates back to the Council Resolution 'A New Approach to technical harmonisation and standards' (1985) and implementing directives. Following the transition to the NLF (Regulation EC No 765/2008 and Regulation EU 2019/1020; Decision No 768/2008/EC) and the 2012 *mise à jour* (COM (2011) 315 final, 1 June 2011, Regulation (EU) 1025/2012), the procedure for adopting harmonised standards is structured in four main phases:

(a) An EU regulatory act defines in deliberately generic terms the essential safety and effectiveness requirements for a product to circulate in the single market: for example, stating that manufactures of AI-MDs must integrate 'appropriate' risk management measures into the production process (see in particular the rules collected in Chapter 3, Section 2: Requirements for High-Risk AI Systems, AI Act);
(b) The Commission makes a formal request (mandate) to the ESOs, aimed at developing the relevant harmonised standards, specifying the essential requirements that the standard must translate into technical specifications: in our case, identifying and describing the 'appropriate' risk management measures for AI-MDs;
(c) Standardisation bodies develop the required technical specifications, which are published as harmonised standards. In the implementation of Art. 40 AI Act, in May 2023, the European Commission made a formal standardisation request to a Joint Technical Committee formed by CEN and CENELEC (JTC 21), in which representatives of industry, civil society, and international standardisation bodies participate as mere observers. JTC 21, whose original deadline of April 2025 has been extended twice, has meanwhile published a list of officially adopted standards, including CEN/CLC ISO/IEC TR 24027:2023 (assessing bias) and ISO/IEC 23894:2023 (risk management);
(d) Harmonised standards, published in the Official Journal of the European Union (OJEU) and adopted by national standardisation bodies, integrate the essential safety requirements identified by the respective sectoral regulations.

2.3 The Fiction of Consensus and the 'Meroni' Doctrine

In short, harmonised standardisation carries out the non-legislative task of making *Blankettnormen* more specific through technical specifications produced by private entities. This conflicts with the limits imposed on the delegation of 'rule-making powers' since the Meroni case (Case 10/56, Meroni, [1958] ECR 1958). This view is consistent with the Court of Justice's jurisprudence, set out in the James Elliott case (CJEU C-613/14—James Elliott Construction), which established that technical standards form an integral part of 'Union law' and are therefore indirectly subject to judicial review under Art. 267 TFEU (see also: CJEU C-160/20 Stichting Rookpreventie Jeugd v Staatssecretaris van Volksgezondheid, Welzijn en Sport; C-630/16, Anstar; C-185/17, SAKSA; C-475/19 P and C-688/19 P, Germany/Commission).

Irrespective of the nature of standardisation—whether regulatory or merely executive—the integration of harmonised standards into sectoral rules presents manufacturers with a dilemma: either implement the 'essential requirements' needed for the marketing of a product independently, demonstrating that they guarantee at least equivalent performance, or adopt the harmonised standard and benefit from the 'presumption of conformity' of the product with the sectoral rules (Art.

3(2) of Directive 2001/95/EC, Art. 2 of Regulation 1025/2012). However, this is a purely theoretical choice: 'administrative difficulties' and 'additional costs' render the alternative procedure to adopting the standard 'of little or no practical use' (CJEU, C-171/11, Fra. Bo, para. 29). Nevertheless, the fiction of free choice serves to affirm the purely private nature of harmonised standards, the repeated assertion of copyright over them. It also sustains the ideological representation of the private co-regulation as consensual and participatory—all of which is increasingly problematic in light of the CJEU's decision C-588/21 P—Public.Resource.Org.

The normative relevance of standardisation is rooted in the private enforcement procedure known as conformity assessment, which is contingent on the intended use indicated by the manufacturer in relation to binding parameters. In Regulations (EU) 2017/745 (medical devices) and 2017/746 (in vitro diagnostic medical devices), hereafter referred to as MDRs, the classification of a device into one of three main risk classes is determined by the combination of its intended clinical use with a series of objective parameters (e.g. duration of body contact, invasiveness, and need for an external energy source). Each risk class is associated with a specific conformity assessment procedure. In short, products in the first risk class require only a self-assessment by the manufacturer. By contrast, products in the moderate (Class I m, s, r; Class IIa) and high (Class IIb and Class III) risk classes require a conformity assessment by an independent professional entity (notified body). The manufacturer selects this entity from a list accredited by national authorities and the European Commission. In the event of a favourable outcome, a declaration formulated by the manufacturer and certified by the notified body is issued, thereby reporting the standards that have been used and permitting the product to circulate within the single market. Software integrated into a hardware medical device is subject to the same classification as the primary device. However, if the software is designed and used as an independent device (Software as a Medical Device, or SaMD), different classification rules apply.

3 Artificial Intelligence as a Medical Device

3.1 Classification of AI-MDs in the AI Act-MDR System

The analysis of the conformity assessment procedure demonstrates that technical standardisation has evolved into a realm where the choices relative to the balance between innovation and safety are actually made.

Art. 6 AI Act classifies high-risk AI systems into two distinct categories. The first category (Art. 6(1)) includes systems that are intended to be used as safety components of a product or that are products themselves. These systems are subject to harmonisation legislation based on the New Legislative Framework listed in Annex I, and they are also required to undergo conformity assessment in order to be placed on the market or put into service. The second category (Art. 6(2)) covers systems intended for use in one of the eight strategic sectors defined in Annex III. These systems are used to implement identification and control and access authorisation over essential services and functions operated by public or private authorities (Annex III).

Artificial intelligence-based medical devices meet both conditions for inclusion in the first category. In other words, all AI-MDs will be classified as 'high risk' according to Art. 6(1) AI Act and, consequently, will be subject to conformity assessment in accordance with the MDRs and additional requirements identified in Art. 43.3 AI Act.

Manufacturers can integrate their quality management system into the conformity assessment devised by the MDRs (Art. 8(2), 9 and 17) and produce unified, standardised technical documentation (Art. 11). In particular, classification rule no. 11 of Annex VIII to the MDRs applies. This states that software intended for diagnosis, therapy, or monitoring falls into Risk Class IIa unless it is likely to cause death, irreversible deterioration of the patient's condition, serious deterioration, or the need for surgical intervention. Otherwise, it falls into Risk Classes III and IIb (the latter also applicable to vital parameter monitoring devices).

3.2 The Problem of **Continuous** *Algorithms and the Innovation/Safety Trade-Off*

Applying harmonised standards to medical devices can affect technological development. As machine learning (ML) systems learn and self-correct, their performance improves over time. ML-based devices differ according to whether the algorithm used is 'discrete' (Adaptive Discrete Improvement Algorithms, or ADI) or 'continuous' (Adaptive Continuous Learning Algorithms, or ACL). In discrete mode (ADI), the system is periodically retrained by the manufacturer based on new datasets, and products are released to the market in a new version after each training cycle. In continuous mode (ACL), the learning phase is performed automatically by the system. Even before the AI Act came into effect, the emergence of ACL algorithms meant that products are frozen at the time of market entry, as they could evolve in such a way as to no longer have the same performance and safety characteristics for which they were approved. Moreover, over time, two identical products supplied to two different users may exhibit divergent behaviours depending on inputs.

The AI Act has maintained this precautionary approach. According to Art. 43(4) (Conformity Assessment), any system undergoing a 'substantial modification' must undergo the conformity assessment procedure again. This obligation applies to modifications identified by the manufacturer as predetermined in the technical documentation, as well as to solutions aimed at ensuring compliance with the essential requirements for high-risk AI systems (Annex IV, 2(f)). The resilience of the precautionary approach is a prime example of the innovation/safety trade-off that dominates public discourse on technology regulation. The exclusion of products in continuous mode is likely to hinder the development of more efficient and innovative devices. Conversely, favouring the precautionary principle is consistent with including medical devices in the category of high-risk systems. This is determined by the applicability of the conformity assessment procedures provided for each sector by the corresponding product safety regulations, whose primary purpose is to protect human health and physical integrity. This tension between innovation and safety provides the context for analysing liability rules in this sector.

4 Toward Complementarity Between Safety Rules and Liability Rules

4.1 The Institutional Design

In risk societies, zero risk does not exist. No quality or risk management system can guarantee the clinical efficacy or long-term safety of a medical device with absolute certainty; even if it were feasible, such a guarantee would likely stifle technological innovation beyond what is socially desirable. Nevertheless, the impact on victims of innovation justifies the imposition of an obligation on 'manufacturers' (as defined by sectoral regulations) to compensate for harm caused by products that conform to safety standards. 'Manufacturers shall [...] have measures in place to provide sufficient financial coverage in respect of their potential liability under Directive 85/374/EEC, without prejudice to more protective measures under national law' (Art. 10(16), MDRs). The principle of separation between safety rules and liability rules is reiterated in the AI Act (recitals 9 and 10, and Art. 2), which states that 'all rights and remedies [...] including as regards the compensation of possible damages pursuant to Council Directive 85/374/EEC, remain unaffected and fully applicable'. This should dispel any residual doubt that compliance with standards constitutes a defence. 'Risk' and 'defect' are distinct normative concepts. At the same time, the existence of an institutional design combining ex ante supervision and ex post compensation justifies a contextual approach based on a directive of complementarity between safety rules and liability rules.

From a coordination perspective, the issue is how to distribute responsibility among the various actors in the technological-health ecosystem, with the objective of avoiding an excessive burden on clinical personnel while promoting the safe integration of artificial intelligence into medical practice. It is evident that the opacity and complexity of ML systems constitute an objective impediment to the implementation of a proof-of-defect-based discipline within the framework of the product liability model introduced by Directive 85/374/EEC and reiterated by Directive (EU) 2024/2853. This is particularly relevant where the system in question involves intricate interactions between different subjects that are accountable to different liability regimes. This is the case of medical devices, wherein clinical personnel, healthcare organisations, manufacturers, and operators can be deemed liable in varying capacities.

4.2 *The Limits of Product Liability: The Case of False Negative Diagnosis*

From this point of view, the paradigmatic case of an imaging diagnostic system producing a false negative that goes undetected by the medical team poses an epistemic problem that extends beyond the search for optimal coordination between product liability regimes and product safety regulations. Provided the system remains within the margin of error certified by the manufacturer, a single erroneous result can be considered neither the outcome of defective functioning under the product liability directives nor a performance that exceeds the permitted risk threshold under the medical device regulations. As AI-MDs are statistical systems, their performance must also be assessed statistically. Conversely, critically evaluating the results produced by the diagnostic system is a medical service that requires organisations using the system to employ suitably specialised and trained medical staff. Therefore, any harm suffered by the patient is not the result of a defect in the AI-MD, but rather an error in the medical service provided—namely, an incorrect diagnosis.

Yet, this argument does not necessarily imply that liability based on medical malpractice is the most appropriate solution. In fact the risk of doctors relying too heavily on AI-MDs is symptomatic of a larger issue: medical practice, organised as a complex network of services and professional relationships, creates conditions conducive to systemic errors, where human error becomes a link in a chain of causes. Attributing liability to the organisation that employs professionals, along the lines of vicarious liability or according to the model applied in Italy by Law 24/2017, is a more balanced solution. This approach attributes liability to the entity best equipped to prevent harm, while also introducing a corrective measure to address the issue of defensive medicine in connection with the use of AI-MDs.

The conclusion may differ if the current restrictions on using ML systems in 'continuous' mode were removed in the future (above, 3.2). In this scenario, the inherent complexity of the AI-MDs, combined with the rule limiting liability at the time the system is placed on the market, and the development risk defence, would ultimately shift liability actions towards doctors and healthcare facilities. Directive (EU) 2024/2853 acknowledges this possibility by establishing a presumption of defect based on product complexity. This includes 'innovative medical devices' and the 'complex nature of the technology used, such as machine learning', as well as a causal link that would require the claimant 'to explain the inner workings of an AI system' (see recital 48 and Art. 10(4)). The extension of liability if the defect 'comes into being after that moment as a result of software or related services within their control, be it in the form of updates, upgrades or machine-learning algorithms' (see recital 50 and Art. 11(2)) moves in the same direction, as does the possibility for Member States to derogate from the 'development risk defence' (see recital 59 and Art. 18(1)).

5 Three Trends and a Policy Proposal

From a systematic perspective, three emerging trends merit attention.

The first trend relates to the relationship between the AI Act and sectoral regulations. It has effectively been stated that artificial intelligence 'does not exist' as a coherent and unitary legal category [3]. In light of the results of this paper, this observation can be refined—and to some extent corrected—by noting that there is no comprehensive, self-contained *regulation* specifically addressing artificial intelligence. This is particularly evident in the case of high-risk systems, where the AI Act establishes general principles (such as transparency, robustness, and human oversight) and cross-cutting rules (such as general conformity requirements, documentation and transparency obligations, and conformity assessment procedures), leaving to sectoral legislation and technical standards the task of implementing rules that account for specific contexts and needs.

The second trend relates to the exhaustion of the long century of civil liability, i.e. the end of the great cycle of liability expansion that accompanied the emergence of risk society. Product safety legislation and liability rules can be seen as communicating vessels: as the former increases, the latter reduces, particularly with regard to the general preventive (deterrent) and redistributive functions of the costs of accidents associated with mass industrial production. Civil liability, so to speak, 'returns home' to its compensatory function—but this return is conditional on the availability of adequate standardisation procedures and updated technical standards.

This introduces the third trend. The return to the compensatory dimension does not imply a return to a depoliticised view of liability that is divorced from the economic and social context. This perspective is ruled out, among other things, by the reference to liability rules in the AI Act and in the MDRs, and even more so by the fact that under Art. 6(1) and Annex I of the AI Act, safety rules and technical standards form part of a structurally (and deliberately) incomplete regulatory framework. Consequently, the task of standardisation bodies will become ever more strategic and sensitive.

The last point suggests that the reasons given in the past for revising the NLF to make ESOs more accountable and open to the participation of active stakeholders are even more compelling in the context of the digital economy. At a minimum, such a revision should ensure active participation of associations representing civil society and consumer groups in standardisation procedures, mandate due diligence requirements for ESOs, introduce mandatory reviews (sunset rules) for high-risk standards, and extend civil liability to ESOs in the event of damage caused by products that conform to inadequate or outdated standards.

Bibliography

1. Castronovo C (2015) Eclissi del diritto civile. Giuffrè, Milano
2. Schepel H (2005) The constitution of private governance. Hart Publishing, Oxford
3. Bertolini A (2022) Artificial intelligence does not exist! Defying the technology-neutrality narrative in the regulation of civil liability for advanced technologies. Eur Dirit Priv 2:369–420
4. Al Mureden E (2019) Product safety e product liability nella prospettiva del danno da prodotto conforme. In: Alpa G (ed) La responsabilità del produttore. Giuffrè, Milano, pp 515–537
5. Almada M, Petit N (2025) The EU AI Act: between the rock of product safety and the hard place of fundamental rights. Common Market Law Rev 62:85–120
6. Bertolini A (2024) Intelligenza Artificiale e Responsabilità civile. Problema, sistema, funzioni. Il Mulino, Bologna
7. Bonatti A et al (2025) Artificial intelligence in healthcare. In: Calderai V, De Maria C (eds) The regulation of health technologies: a European perspective. Pisa University Press, Pisa, pp 213–252
8. Cafaggi F (2008) Product safety, private standard setting and information networks. EUI working paper law no. 17. https://ssrn.com/abstract=1303419
9. Cafaggi F, Watt MH (eds) (2009) The regulatory function of European private law. Edward Elgar, Cheltenham
10. Calabresi G (1970) The costs of accidents. A legal and economical analysis. Yale University Press, New Haven
11. Calabresi G (1985) Ideals, beliefs, attitudes, and the law. Syracuse University Press, Syracuse
12. Cauffman C, Eliantonio M (2020) The legitimacy of standardisation as a regulatory technique. A. Cross-disciplinary and multi-level analysis. Edward Elgar, Cheltenham
13. Chiti E (2022) Normalizzazione. In: Enciclopedia del Diritto. I Tematici, vol III. Giuffrè, Milano
14. Cuccuru P. (2019) Interest representation in European standardisation: the case of CEN and CENELEC. Amsterdam Law School Research Paper No. 2019–52. https://ssrn.com/abstract=3505290
15. D'Adda A (2022) Danni "da robot" (specie in ambito sanitario) e pluralità di responsabili tra sistema della responsabilità civile ed iniziative di diritto europeo. Rivista di diritto civile 68:805–837
16. Ebers M (2022) Standardizing AI. The case of the European Commission proposal for an "artificial intelligence act". In: Dimatteo LA, Poncibò C, Cannarsa M (eds) The Cambridge handbook of artificial intelligence. Global perspectives on law and ethics. Cambridge University Press, Cambridge, pp 321–342
17. Fusaro A (2019) I prodotti difettosi e pericolosi: le responsabilità. In: Alpa G (ed) La responsabilità del produttore. Giuffrè, Milano, pp 361–384
18. Gérardy M (2022) The use of copyrighted technical standards in the operationalisation of European Union law: the status quo position of the general court in Public.Resource.Org (T-185/19). Eur J Risk Regul 13(3):532–37. https://doi.org/10.1017/err.2022.16
19. Lundqvist B (2017) European harmonised standards, EU law and copyright. Faculty of Law, Stockholm University Research Paper No. 11. https://ssrn.com/abstract=2981338
20. Maliha G, Gerke S, Cohen IG, Parikh RB (2021) Artificial intelligence and liability in medicine: balancing safety and innovation. Milbank Q 99(3):629–647. https://doi.org/10.1111/1468-0009.12504
21. Micklitz HW (2023) The role of standards in future EU digital policy legislation. A consumer perspective. ANEC-BEUC legal study, BEUC, Brussels
22. Morello F, Coro F, Calderai V (2025) Liability for malfunctioning medical devices. In: Calderai V, De Maria C (eds) The regulation of health technologies: a European perspective. Pisa University Press, Pisa, pp 97–124
23. Palmerini E (2025) La governance dei sistemi ad alto rischio nell' Artificial Intelligence Act: Uno Sguardo Panoramico. Foro Ital V:35–48

24. Resta G (2022) Cosa c'è di 'europeo' nella proposta di regolamento Ue sull'intelligenza artificiale? Diritto dell'informazione e dell'informatica 38:340–367
25. Soroiu A (2024) The fall of the great paywall for EU harmonised standards: the CJEU dismantles EU standardisation in C-588/21 P (public.Resource.Org). VerfBlog. https://verfassungsblog.de/eu-harmonised-standards/. https://doi.org/10.59704/5a60ea5d42c2b059
26. Tovo C (2018) Judicial review of harmonized standards: changing the paradigms of legality and legitimacy of private rulemaking under EU law. Common Market Law Rev 55(4):1145–1184
27. Van Gestel R, Micklitz HW (2013) European integration through standardization: how judicial review is breaking down the club house of private standardization bodies. Common Market Law Rev 50:145–182
28. Van Leeuwen B (2017) European standardisation of services and its impact on private law. In: Paradoxes of convergence. Hart Publishing, Portland
29. Van Leeuwen B (2019) Market access, the new approach and private law. Eur Rev Private Law 27(2):269–292
30. Verbruggen P (2019) Good governance of private standardization and the role of tort law. Eur Rev Priv Law 27(2):319–352
31. Volpato A (2017) The harmonized standards before the ECJ: James Elliot construction. Common Market Law Rev 54:591–604

Chapter 10
AI and Medical Liability

Mirko Faccioli

1 Introduction

At a global level, advanced robotics and Artificial Intelligence (henceforth, AI) are already used in various medical settings, ranging from diagnosis and medical treatment to surgery, with sector-specific applications, such as radiology or virology. AI medical tools are particularly suitable for carrying out high-precision surgical procedures or even personalized assistance tasks. When AI supports healthcare decisions, there is a significant decrease in diagnostic times and medical errors.

In addition, it should be emphasized that by increasing the quality and efficiency of treatments, the use of AI in healthcare is capable of producing considerable positive economic returns since it significantly diminishes the costs incurred by both the national health service to perform medical services and the population to benefit from them. In fact, several AI applications may help national health systems to decrease waiting times for specialist exams dramatically, travel between home and hospital facilities, or prevent people from going to hospital emergency rooms for unnecessary reasons.

Many initiatives have been undertaken by the European Union (EU) in the last few years to advance the development and uptake of AI technologies, to help EU citizens better monitor their health, receive better diagnoses and more personalized treatments, as well as live healthier lives. Nevertheless, the current situation in the EU indicates that healthcare organizations are still slow in implementing AI technologies in healthcare and that the level of adoption is low overall. The underuse of technology triggers what economists call "opportunity costs", which in this context is the difference in productivity and quality gains of an AI-supported health system

M. Faccioli (✉)
University of Verona, Verona, Italy
e-mail: mirko.faccioli@univr.it

A. Bernes, S. Thobani (eds.), *Digitalisation in Health Care between New Technologies, Data and Research*, Services and Business Process Reengineering, https://doi.org/10.1007/978-981-95-6982-3_10

and one that does not use or does not use AI enough, minus the cost for purchasing and maintaining the technology.

What certainly plays a key role in this situation, especially when considering that there is essentially no case law on medical malpractice involving AI, is the current lack of legal clarity with regard to the civil liability that could arise in this field. This uncertainty is a consequence of the main AI-related characteristics: (1) the capacity to operate autonomously, that is, without human supervision or with limited human supervision; (2) the opacity, namely the fact that algorithms often no longer come as more or less easily readable code, but as a "black-box" that has evolved through self-learning and can be verified as to its effects, but not entirely understood as to its proceedings; (3) the unpredictability, namely the fact that it is often impossible to precisely and consistently predict what specific actions an intelligent system will take to achieve its objectives, even if its terminal goals are known.

In this scenario and in light of existing rules on medical negligence and product liability, it is actually hard to determine how civil liability for damage suffered by the patient might be apportioned between the medical practitioner, the hospital that decides to adopt the AI-based solution and/or employs the practitioner, and the manufacturer and the programmer of the machine. This latter topic, although, is of a general nature and, to a large extent, goes beyond the specifics of the health sector; therefore, it will not be discussed in detail in this paper.

The abovementioned legal uncertainty, on the one hand, discourages physicians and hospitals from buying and employing AI-based systems, and, on the other hand, disincentivizes manufacturing companies from investing in research and development related to this field.

Due to this situation, it also seems likely that doctors will tend to adopt defensive medicine practices and decision-making, i.e., recommending a diagnostic test or medical treatment that is not necessarily the best option for the patient, but that mainly serves to protect the physician against possible subsequent claims for damages. The issue of defensive medicine is particularly pronounced in this field compared to the broader context of medical malpractice. The use of advanced technological solutions can heighten patient expectations, which may lead to increased frustration if treatments prove ineffective or harmful. This frustration can, in turn, drive patients to seek compensation.

To promote the expansion of AI in medicine, it is therefore essential, before accidents happen, to investigate the civil liability arising from the use of this technology, bringing the clarity needed to foster research and development. In other words, it is necessary to ascertain whether the issues raised by the use of AI can be faced by applying the current legal and case-law framework on medical malpractice, or whether a legislative reform of the subject matter is required.

In doing so, it must be pointed out that the autonomy, opacity, and unpredictability of AI systems raise the difficulty of achieving a satisfactory trade-off between two different exigencies. On the one hand, those characteristics should play a role in reconstructing the liability regime of health care providers; otherwise, they would be discouraged from adopting AI, with all its benefits, because of the concern of being held responsible for events and incidents beyond their control. On the other hand, proper attention should be given to the consideration that the patient, injured by an AI system, should benefit from no less protection than that usually enjoyed by patients injured by healthcare treatment carried out using traditional methods. Failing that, the trust in AI necessary for this technology to spread widely will never develop in society.

It must be highlighted that these issues could not be tackled simply by attributing (some) new form of legal capacity to AI systems ("e-person"). Although fascinating, also for historical reasons, this approach has already been amply demonstrated to be theoretically inadmissible and of little practical use, especially when referring to the area of civil liability.

At an introductory level, it must be finally considered that, although terminology and boundaries differ, virtually all legal European systems differentiate between contractual and forms of extra-contractual liability. In the field of medical malpractice, most European Member States allow claimants to choose whether to base their claim on delict or contract, so that non-contractual liabilities generally compete with liability claims in contract.

2 The Nature of Healthcare Obligation and the Physician's Individual Liability

The first legal question raised by the use of AI involves the qualification of the medical activity within the dichotomy between obligations "of means" (or "of conduct") and obligations "of result".

The activity at issue is generally considered the paradigmatic example of the first type of obligation, due to the random nature of medical science and the unpredictable reactions of the human body. Nevertheless, in some cases, judgements have claimed that it is possible to recognize an obligation of result on the part of the doctor. The basic idea is that the performance of certain healthcare treatments is presided over by specific and highly binding technical rules, to the point that a close link can be established, also with the support of statistical data, on the one hand, between the compliance with those rules and the achievement of a certain clinical outcome, and, on the other hand, between the failure of the treatment and an error in the performance.

However, even though AI may vastly increase the accuracy and effectiveness of medical intervention, it does not appear that its use automatically requires the development of such reasoning, disregarding the circumstances of the concrete case. On the contrary, the use of AI constitutes a neutral factor concerning the qualification of the nature of the medical performance, which, in the absence of additional elements leading to the contrary, should normally fall, according to the general tendency highlighted above, within the scope of obligations of means and not of result.

Consequently, liability for non-fulfilment of the clinical performance is subject to the criterion of fault, parametrized on the professional diligence and in compliance with the guidelines and good practices in the field of medical science. From the point of view of fault-based liability, it must then be excluded that the doctor can be held liable for an AI system malfunctioning outside the scope of their control due to its high degree of autonomy and opacity. The physician's liability is limited to cases where the damage resulted from the incorrect use of the machine due to negligence. By way of example, medical professionals may be held liable for using AI without having the necessary skills, for having used an intelligent system knowing or negligently ignoring its defectiveness, for not having detected the wrongness of the instructions provided by the machine to the extent that it was detectable by diligent verification, or for having used such technologies to deal with a clinical case whose specificities required the use of traditional treatment methods. Surgeons in particular must maintain their traditional surgical skills in order to minimize potential damage when robotic and computerized systems inevitably fail. At some point, the standard of care may shift to postponing the procedure until the robot is repaired, rather than risking complications by performing the procedure in a manner with which they are only somewhat familiar. This situation can become problematic if the surgeon has rarely, if ever, performed the procedure without the assistance of a robot.

However, a part of the literature has suggested contrary solutions, based on the discipline of special types of non-contractual strict liability. Applying this regime to the case of AI would mean that liability is imposed on physicians, not because of their own wrongful act, but due to their relationship with the "tortfeasor" AI system. These approaches vary extensively.

Some argue that humans and AI could be, respectively, assimilated, by way of analogy and in the light of the so-called vicarious liability, to parents and children, to preceptor and pupil, to principal and employee, or even to owner and animal. The main argument of this theory is that no one should be able to exclude the attribution provided for by vicarious liability provisions simply by employing technical means of support instead of human helpers. However, the rules on vicarious liability have been conceived and tailored to the characteristics of natural intelligence, human or at most animal. Therefore, they cannot be fruitfully transposed to the context of AI, either directly or by analogy.

Equally unconvincing is the reconduction of medical services performed through AI under the strict liability regime that some jurisdictions provide for in respect of damage caused by dangerous activities. Already controversial in general terms, the qualification of medical activity as "dangerous" appears completely implausible in our case, where it is associated with the use of advanced technological solutions, capable of vastly increasing the safety of treatments.

At first sight, the thesis that considers applicable in the field of AI the strict liability regime for damage caused by things in one's custody (or control), first developed in France but later also adopted by several other European countries, could seem more reliable. However, this too can be contested: even an extensive interpretation of these rules maintains the perspective of human control over the thing, which appears incompatible with the level of technology and the degree of autonomy and unpredictability of AI-driven machines.

Another objection that can be made against all the aforementioned theories is based on the phenomenon of defensive medicine. It must be borne in mind that a fault-based liability for physicians has been elaborated by scholars, and in some countries (for example, Italy) also expressly confirmed by lawmakers, with the aim of relieving the judicial pressure on medical personnel and countering the aforementioned phenomenon. Hence, these purposes cannot be hindered by rendering the doctor's liability regime more rigid by way of interpretation.

Lastly, it must be considered that strict liability is generally applied in cases of unforeseeable events to date and that the definition of harm from AI as an unforeseeable event remains uncertain. A further limitation is the economic impact that such a measure would entail, as many litigations would result in compensations even in the burden-of-proof absence.

3 The Liability of the Hospital

The liability regime of medical practitioners described above does not result in a gap in protection for the patient harmed by the malfunctioning of the AI system used in treatment, since the patient may usefully bring a claim for damages against the healthcare facility. The latter can always be subject, in addition to (and even apart from) indirect liability for the conduct of the medical staff, to direct and independent liability for the so-called organizational defect that arises from the breach of the obligation, deriving from the healthcare contract concluded with patients, to provide an organizational context of an adequate level in which to receive them.

In this scenario, the hospital must submit its technical equipment to general periodic control and maintenance procedures, and to ad hoc checks before each concrete use, its liability being excluded only for damages linked to manufacturing and operational defects that cannot be detected through diligent inspection. It is important to emphasize that, since the hospital's organizational duties fall within the sphere of obligations of result, the liability arising from their non-fulfilment is assessed by employing, instead of the criterion of fault used to test the individual liability of the physician, a more rigorous parameter of an objective nature, which ends up placing the risk of non-fulfilment deriving from all the failures that may occur within its organizational framework on the healthcare facility, with the only limit of the unexpected impossibility not attributable to the hospital.

In our field of interest, these principles lead to recognizing the liability of the healthcare facility for damage caused by AI systems that have not undergone the checks and maintenance and updating procedures necessary to ensure their regular functioning. On the other hand, the hospital should not be held liable for damage caused by a defect in the AI systems that can be ascribed to the device's construction and implementation phase and that cannot be detected by diligent examination, in which case the sole liability of those who took part in the manufacture and setting up of the machine would be relevant. However, from the point of view of strict liability for organizational defect, the circumstance must be proved by the healthcare facility. Otherwise, it must compensate for the damage suffered by the patient subjected to the treatment carried out employing the malfunctioning IA system.

In addition, the healthcare facility could be blamed for having assigned to the use of AI systems personnel lacking the knowledge, skills, and training necessary to properly use intelligent machines or for not having implemented procedures designed to mitigate risks associated with the AI.

Based on the abundant case law on the subject of liability for instrumental deficiencies of healthcare facilities, in the future, the latter may also be held liable for not having purchased and employed innovative technical tools, such as intelligent machines based on algorithms, which are considered safe and have been widely adopted in the national healthcare system. From this point of view, it must also be considered that early adopters risk stepping outside the standard of care when other hospitals are reluctant to embrace new AI-powered technologies, whereas late adopters also risk violating the standard of care if they fail to adopt beneficial AI that most other facilities have already accepted.

4 The Causal Nexus

As in all medical malpractice liability actions, the claim brought by the patient damaged by AI must also deal with issues relating to the causal nexus, the reconstruction of which may indeed be particularly complex in our subject matter, given the opacity, autonomy, and unpredictability of AI systems. In other words, difficulties may well arise in establishing whether or not the harm suffered by the patient was caused by a malfunction of the intelligent machine. From this point of view, it must also be borne in mind that, despite its impressive performance in diagnosis, prognosis, and image analysis, autonomous medical AI technology has important limitations, and cannot yet distinguish between causation and correlation, engage in conceptual thinking, demonstrate human common sense, or analyse information across several knowledge domains.

However, what thus comes to the surface is not a new issue. The evidentiary problem of the unknown cause in medical liability has been studied in great depth in recent years. In fact, according to some scholars, the problem has probably less to do with AI than with the fact that establishing liability is always a complex issue when medical treatments are at stake. The main reason for that, though not the only one, is the difficulty in assessing causation when the functioning of the human body is involved.

In any case, it seems especially interesting to report the solution practised in the Italian legal system, where the issue at stake has been solved by establishing two major rules. The patient is required to prove the material causal link between the doctor's conduct and the harmful event, consisting of the harm to health or the aggravation of the pathological situation, or the onset of a new illness. Whereas, where the patient has proved the aforementioned material causal nexus, it is the other party's burden to prove that they have accurately performed the medical treatment or that its failure was due to an impossibility resulting from an unattributable cause. Therefore, if the cause of the harm suffered by the patient remains unknown, the patient will suffer the consequences of having their action dismissed. In contrast, if the reason that prevented the doctors and the hospital from correctly performing the medical service remains unknown, the latter will bear the costs by way of paying damages.

It is furthermore important to mention that, more generally in Europe, there are several situations in which the patient's burden of proof is either relaxed or shifts completely to the defendant. For example, the burden of proof on causation might shift to the doctors and the hospital if the device or system involved is deemed to be in the defendant's sphere of control, if the defendant is in a better position than the patient to bear the burden of proof, or in case of "gross errors" committed by the healthcare providers.

In addition, healthcare providers using AI to treat patients may assert defences of contributory and comparative fault, which can reduce or eliminate the defendant's liability when the plaintiff's or another party's negligence caused or contributed to the plaintiff's injury. For example, a patient who provides incorrect information might be negligent if the provider used AI that relied on this information to produce a treatment recommendation that the provider later relied upon. Moreover, a third-party AI developer might be negligent if they provided incorrect instructions regarding the use of black-box AI, and the provider relied on those instructions to make a recommendation.

In conclusion, through these principles, it should also be possible to deal, in a way that can be considered satisfying, with the uncertainties surrounding the reconstruction of the aetiological nexus that arise in disputes over damage caused by medical treatment performed with the aid of AI.

5 Informed Consent and Liability for Infringement of the Right to Self-determination of the Patient

To conclude, liability for breach of informed consent may eventually also arise in the area of our interest. Although it is subject to the general regulation on the matter, informed consent to treatment performed using AI presents certain peculiarities for which a reflection is required.

Fundamentally, it is necessary to question whether the physician's duty to inform also includes the use of AI and, if so, how detailed the information to be provided to the patient should be.

This question is positively answered by several scholars, who claim that the physician should provide the patient with the most complete and exhaustive information about the characteristics of the AI system employed in the treatment, in particular by focusing on the degree of autonomy, opacity, and (un)controllability of the machine. However, the existing laws on informed consent in the medical field generally require, following the Codes of Medical Ethics, that the information should be modulated in light of the patient's ability to understand and their moral condition; it is therefore left to the doctors' discretion whether or not to include details of a technical nature among the elements provided to their interlocutor.

From another point of view, about information concerning the possibility of a harmful malfunction of the AI, it must be questioned if the general orientation that limits the content of the physician's obligation to provide information to foreseeable risks only and excludes the need to inform the patient of abnormal and exceptional outcomes, borderline fortuitous, that do not have any relevance according to the *id quod plerumque accidit*, can be applied in this field as well.

However, these aspects will not be discussed further, as they are the focus of a separate essay contained in this volume (C. De Menech, "AI, health and obligations of information").

6 Concluding Remarks

Every generation of legal experts has had to perform the task of investigating the effects that the advent of new technology has had on one or more areas of application of the law. For example, the generation of the early twentieth century investigated the changes brought by the motorization of road traffic on tort law, and the generation of the last part of the twentieth century had to investigate the impact of digitalization on the format of contracts, as well as the violation of copyright law. The current generation, on the other hand, has had to study the extraordinary changes, both positive and negative, that the development of AI seems capable of causing within every area of law.

One of the areas most affected by the progress of AI is health law, owing to the success of AI devices in the medical field. The benefits of medical treatments and scientific developments are, however, accompanied by empirical risks, technical complexity, ethical concerns, and, therefore, legal issues. As is often the case, new problems emerging from the use of AI in healthcare raise the debate on whether modern technology requires new specific legislation or existing legislation and concepts may be adjusted to it.

According to some scholars, the law on redress in health-care practiced through AI should even evolve from an issue of civil liability into one of financial management of losses, pursuant to no-fault redress schemes. Such schemes should apply in cases where there is no evidence that doctors, producers, and programmers of AI devices acted in conditions of negligence, imprudence, or unskillfulness, and their activity appropriately complied with scientifically validated standards. In other cases, traditional civil liability rules would continue to apply and play a role of deterrence.

On the contrary, my opinion is that, in light of today's state of technological evolution, medical civil liability arising from the use of AI should be properly addressed with the current legal and case-law framework on medical malpractice.

The set of duties and responsibilities of physicians and health care facilities dealing with AI systems described so far does not seem to need to be called into question in light of the provisions regarding the obligations of deployers of high-risk A.I. systems provided for in the AI Act, which are certainly also applicable to practitioners and hospitals that should use medical devices that can be classified as such. Without affecting the essence of the medical performance and the organizational duties of health care facilities, these provisions, in fact, principally impose the following: take technical and organizational measures to ensure that such systems are used in accordance with the accompanying instructions; entrust human oversight to persons with the necessary competence, training, and authority; ensure that input data is relevant and sufficiently representative in view of the intended purpose of the system; monitor the operation of the system, suspend its use, and inform providers and relevant authorities in the event of high risks or serious incidents; keep the logs automatically generated by the system that are under their control for a period, appropriate to the purpose of the system, of at least 6 months; where applicable, perform an assessment of the impact on fundamental rights that the use of such system may produce.

Possibly, some minor adjustments by way of interpretation or law reform could be appropriate. For example, it could be stipulated by law that the indications provided by AI are equivalent to the guidelines and good clinical practices with which the physician must comply in the execution of their activity. In this way, the judge would have a solid normative basis to include the doctor's behaviour regarding the response of AI in the judgement.

A more profound review of the current legal system may instead be appropriate, if not necessary, only if and when it will be possible to build machines capable of performing healthcare services in complete autonomy and without human intervention: in other words, in a scenario of "medical-robots", that is something which may not ever really occur.

Bibliography

1. Bertolini A (2020) Artificial intelligence and civil liability. Study requested by the European Parliament's Committee on Legal Affairs, Brussels
2. De Menech C (2022) Artificial intelligence and self-determination in medical field. Eur J Privacy Law Technol 1:164–180
3. Geistfeld MA, Karner E, Koch BA, Wendehorst C (eds) (2023) Civil liability for artificial intelligence and software. De Gruyer, Berlin
4. Karner E (2020) Liability for medical robots and autonomous medical devices. In: Karner E, Spier J, Magnus U, Widmer P (eds) Essays in honour of Helmut Koziol. Jan Sramek Verlag, Wien, pp 57–77
5. Lohsse S, Schulze R, Staudenmayer D (eds.) (2023) Liability for AI. Münster Colloquia on EU Law and Digital Economy VII. Nomos, Baden-Baden
6. Marchisio E (2020) Proposal toward "no-fault" civil liability regulation following artificial intelligence evolution in health-care. MediaLaws 2:153–171

7. Mehta D (2024) The role of artificial intelligence in healthcare and medical negligence. Liverpool Law Rev 45:125–142
8. Pagallo U, O'Sullivan S, Nevejans N et al (2024) The underuse of AI in the health sector: opportunity costs, success stories, risks and recommendations. Health Technol 14:1–14
9. Solaiman B, Cohen IG (eds) (2024) Research handbook on health, AI and the law. Elgar, Cheltenham
10. Sousa Antunes H, Freitas PM, Oliveira AL et al (eds) (2024) Multidisciplinary perspectives on artificial intelligence and the law. Springer, Cham
11. van Kolfschooten H, van Oirschot J (2024) The EU artificial intelligence act (2024): implications for healthcare. Health Policy 149:105–152
12. Voeneky S, Kellmeyer P, Mueller O, Burgad W (eds) (2022) The Cambridge handbook of responsible artificial intelligence. Interdisciplinary perspectives. Cambridge University Press, Cambridge

Chapter 11
AI, Health, and Obligations of Information

Carlotta De Menech

1 AI in Healthcare: Within or Beyond the Scope of Informational Obligations?

The use of artificial intelligence systems in healthcare raises numerous questions that struggle to find adequate answers in positive law, prompting legal experts to suggest evolutionary interpretation or express policy choices while waiting for the legislator to develop the necessary reforms to align the legal framework with technological innovation. Specifically, this chapter addresses the question of whether (and to what extent) the patient must be informed that the diagnosis or therapy proposed by the physician relies on artificial intelligence systems. This issue is currently in a transitional phase. Domestic, supranational, and international law do not include specific rules that explicitly impose on physicians the obligation to involve the patient in the decision to use artificial intelligence (hereinafter, AI) in medical treatment.

However, the problem appears close to a solution through regulatory acts that European and Italian legislators are introducing to govern the rapid spread of AI technologies. In the meantime, legal scholars have a chance to carry out further considerations based on both *ius conditum* and *ius condendum*.

Starting from the current legal framework, we need to consider, first, Art. 32 of the Italian Constitution. The article, read in conjunction with Art. 2 and 13, represents a cornerstone of the constitutional matrix of the principle of self-determination but does not refer to any information that should be given to the patient to ensure the effectiveness of the principle it enshrines. However, the majority of Italian scholars maintain that the article at issue imposes on doctors a duty to provide patients as

C. De Menech (✉)
University of Pavia, Pavia, Italy
e-mail: carlotta.demenech@unipv.it

A. Bernes, S. Thobani (eds.), *Digitalisation in Health Care between New Technologies, Data and Research*, Services and Business Process Reengineering, https://doi.org/10.1007/978-981-95-6982-3_11

much information as possible, including the description of the equipment or technologies that will be employed in the treatment.

The emphasis on medical information stems from a distorted interpretation of Art. 32. In addition to sanctioning the principle of therapeutic self-determination, the constitutional norm

> Protects health as a fundamental right of the individual and in the interest of the community

without establishing a hierarchy between the two values. However, legal experts do not accept the equivalence of health and self-determination, considering that the latter must necessarily prevail over the former. To achieve this outcome, jurists argue that, according to the Constitution of the World Health Organization,

> Health is a state of complete physical, mental, and social well-being and not merely the absence of disease or infirmity.

Consequently, in their view, the notion of health can be assimilated into the individual's perception of the medical treatment and, ultimately, reduced to the personal decision of whether or not to undergo such treatment.

Stripped of its original point of reference (i.e., health in its strict sense), the patient's right to self-determination becomes an absolute power, devoid of limits and substance; or, in other words, a "tyrannical right" when set against other constitutionally protected interests. As necessary to the effective exercise of self-determination, medical information should consequently extend to every detail of the treatment.

In considering this theory, some authors dissent from the majority and argue that the patient's right to health encompasses a broader scope than the right to self-determination. This minority opinion is based on a more complete reading of Art. 32 of the Italian Constitution. By reading this article in its entirety and in considering its constitutional context, it becomes clear that the right to health is closely related to the values of human dignity (Art. 32, par. 2) and the duty of solidarity (Art. 32, par. 2; and Art. 2) and, consequently, has a scope that goes beyond the patient's personal sphere, affecting public protection of health and the social function of medical activity as well.

In connection with these further aspects, the right to health takes on an autonomous meaning and can serve to limit and shape the right to informed consent. In this way, self-determination regains its substance with regard to mental and physical well-being, acknowledging the competences of the doctor as a guide, and the patient's weaknesses as limitations. Conversely, if (in accordance with the majority view) the medical relationship was based only on the patient's will, such a relationship would become of a purely "contractual" nature, and therefore the effectiveness of the patient's right to self-determination could be potentially compromised.

This has been demonstrated in other legal contexts (for example, labour law, consumer law, and banking and financial market law) where the freedom to choose can be diminished because of the weak negotiating position of a contracting party, and consequently some precautions are necessary. For example, rules that adjust the quality and the amount of information on the condition of the fragile party, who may be confused by an explanation which is too detailed.

Moving on to ordinary legislation, we need to consider the Italian Law no. 219 of 22 December 2017 ("Provisions on informed consent and advance treatment directives"), which develops the principle of self-determination in healthcare through specific rules. However, these rules do not clarify whether it is the duty of the doctor to inform the patient or to what extent to inform the patient that the therapy involves AI systems. Specifically, Art. 1, par. 3, of Law no. 219/2017 does not clearly indicate whether the doctor is under a legal obligation to communicate to their patient information about the devices and techniques which will be used in their treatment. Nor can such a content requirement be definitively inferred from the adjectives which the legislator uses in describing the characteristics of the information that must be conveyed to the patient. Indeed, the adjective *complete* seems to suggest full disclosure, whereas the adjective *comprehensible* seems to suggest selecting on the basis of the patient's cognitive and rational skills.

Finally, it must be considered that the need to align the patient's self-determination with their mental condition has also been perceived by some judges in their rulings on healthcare matters. Indeed, Italian courts on occasion consider it necessary to diminish, to a certain extent, the amount of information to be provided to the patient. This is because of their vulnerability and in order to safeguard their health. For instance, several rulings state that doctors must inform the patient about risks typically associated with a treatment, but they must abstain from disclosing abnormal and/or remote risks which do not normally occur in the course of standard medical procedures (see, for example, Cass. 6 Oct. 2021, no. 27112; Cass. 26 May 2020, no. 9706; Cass. 20 May 2016, no. 10414; Cass. 11 Dec. 2013, no. 27751; App. Naples 28 June 2024, no. 2975; and Trib. Milan 2 Sept. 2021, no. 7070). The rationale behind this rule is well explained by some courts (see Cass. 30 July 2004, no. 14638; and similarly, Trib. Bologna 8 August 2005), saying that

> To communicate in addition to the normal risks, abnormal and/or remote risks could instil in the patient an unjustified amount of fear which could discourage them from giving permission for treatment which is both safe and standard in modern medical practice.

2 A Third Way

An approach which avoids information overload for the patient is preferable also in relation to the potential use of AI in healthcare. More precisely, physicians should be allowed to assess whether it is appropriate to communicate to their patients that a diagnosis or therapy involves AI systems. Furthermore, doctors should not be obliged to provide a detailed explanation of the technology at issue.

Such assessments should be made, of course, on a case-by-case basis. Therefore, physicians might reasonably choose to withhold information about the involvement of AI when, after a diligent analysis of the patient, they identify the latter as particularly vulnerable. However, it is worth underlining that the notion of *vulnerability* should not be interpreted in a *categorical* manner, namely as a condition which characterises specific groups, for example, the elderly or individuals with mental disorders (see Cass. 9 September 2024, no. 24124, and Cass. 16 August 2024, no. 22888, which affirms that a patient's decisional autonomy in healthcare cannot be deemed diminished or excluded solely by reason of mental disorders). Rather, vulnerability should be understood in an *ontological* sense, namely as a condition inherent to all human beings which may, however, be intensified by adverse situations in which anyone can find themselves. Consider, for example, patients who suffer severe pain.

On the other hand, some circumstances might reduce, or even remove, the discretion on the part of the physician. For example, if the patient asks specific questions regarding the nature of the tools used in diagnosis or treatment, the doctor should provide truthful answers. Indeed, the physician's duty to satisfy the patient's explicit requests is broader than the general obligation to inform them. This is because, on the one hand, lying is more serious than silence, whereas, on the other hand, doubt is usually a symptom of rationality and competence.

In addition, the nature of the medical treatment may broaden the physician's duty to inform, which can consequently extend to AI systems. For instance, this may occur in the context of cosmetic surgery, where it is generally deemed that the patient must be given more information, since the treatment aims not to safeguard their health, but rather to enhance their physical appearance (see, in this regard, Trib. Reggio Calabria, 1 July 2020, no. 647).

Finally, it must be acknowledged that AI clearly falls within the scope of medical information when such technology manages the operation of a medical device to be used by the patient at home (for example, an AI machine learning model which controls an automated insulin delivery system), or when generative AI systems are involved (for example, a chatbot which is capable of issuing diagnoses or therapeutic advice in natural language). In such cases, the patient interacts directly with the AI system without the contribution of an expert and, therefore, withholding information about the role of the technology could jeoparadise not only the patient's self-determination but the proper course of treatment itself, and thus the patient's health.

For the reasons explained above, a flexible and realistic approach to the data aimed at medical consent would be preferable. In particular, the choice of communicating technical details should be at the discretion of the doctor, who should be permitted to make choices based on reasonableness. Therefore, the doctor makes a decision that does not adhere ideologically to only one of the contrasting values: self-determination and health. Instead, the doctor makes a decision by weighing the patient's right to self-determination against the medical needs arising in a specific situation. Such an approach is necessary to prevent the outcome of the communication of too much information affecting both the patient's self-determination and health. However, such an approach faces the dominant current opinion among legal scholars, who uphold the doctrine of informed consent and, therefore, maintain that physicians must always inform their patients about the AI systems involved in diagnosis or treatment.

3 The Way Chosen by the European Legislator in the AI Act

As I have been highlighting above, the majority of Italian jurists privilege the right to self-determination, thus disregarding other conflicting interests. Moreover, the mainstream opinion appears to be little aware of reality. First, it aims to refine the model of informed consent as it is imagined in legal theory, without accounting for the significant gap between that paradigm and its actual implementation in healthcare experience. Second, the opinion at issue overlooks the fact that most physicians lack the knowledge which would be necessary to explain to patients the functioning of the AI systems involved in medical treatment.

Instead, the European legislator appears to be fully aware of such a deficit. Indeed, Regulation EU/2024/1689 on artificial intelligence (hereinafter, the AI Act) outlines a path, which begins with the adoption of measures aimed at ensuring a sufficient level of AI literacy for all subjects who make use of this technology, including healthcare professionals and, only then, may lead to imposing upon physicians the obligation to inform patients that AI will be used in the diagnosis or therapy.

Indeed, on the one hand, Art. 4 of the AI Act states that

> Providers and deployers of AI systems shall take measures to ensure, to their best extent, a sufficient level of AI literacy of their staff and other persons dealing with the operation and use of AI systems on their behalf, taking onto account their technical knowledge, experience, education and training and the context the AI systems are to be used in, and considering the persons or groups of persons on whom the AI systems are to be used.

This article is a general provision which should already apply from 2 February 2025 (according to Recital 179).

On the other hand, the EU regulation contains some provisions which should apply from 2 August 2026 (according to Recital 179), which may support the inclusion of AI within the scope of healthcare information obligations. Among the provisions under consideration, the clearest one is Recital 93, where the legislator states that

> Deployers of high-risk AI systems [...] play a critical role in informing natural persons and should, when they make decisions or assist in making decisions related natural persons, where applicable, inform the natural persons that they are subject to the use of the high-risk AI system,

specifying that

> This information should include the intended purpose and the type of decisions it makes.

Moving on to the binding provisions of the regulation, no similarly explicit statements can be identified. Consider, firstly, Art. 50, par. 1, of the AI Act (entitled "Transparency obligations for providers and deployers of certain AI systems"), which states that

> Providers shall ensure that AI systems intended to interact directly with natural persons are designed and developed in such a way that the natural persons concerned are informed that they are interacting with an AI system [...].

From this article, it is logical to deduce an "informational duty" of providers toward healthcare professionals (who, indeed, "*interact directly with*" AI systems). Instead, it is not at all evident that the rule imposes an "informational duty" of physicians toward their patients.

Another provision, which is relevant to the issue at stake, is Art. 61, which links the requirement to obtain informed consent from the data subject to the testing of high-risk AI systems in real-world conditions (i.e. outside of so-called regulatory sandboxes). Such a provision does not provide unequivocal indications. Indeed, on the one hand, Art. 61 might be interpreted as supporting a general tendency of the European legislator to favour uses of AI grounded in the explicit will of persons who are subject to the system's decisions or actions. On the other hand, one might conclude that the specific prescription contained in Art. 61 implies that informed consent is not required when AI is used in contexts other than those explicitly contemplated by the provision.

4 The Way Planned by the Italian Legislator

Turning to the Italian legal system, particular attention should be given to the Italian Law no. 132 of 23 September 2025 ("Law on Artificial Intelligence": hereinafter, the "*Law on AI*"). Although they may appear similar, the European approach to the problem at issue and the one chosen at the national level are quite different.

Firstly, Art. 7, par. 3, of the *Law on AI* immediately imposes on the physician the duty to inform the patient that the medical treatment will be performed using AI systems, while Art. 24 postpones the regulation and implementation of programs aimed at providing healthcare workers with at least a basic knowledge of AI technology. In this regard, the latter article indicates the need to develop literacy and training pathways for professionals and workers in the specific sector concerning the use of AI systems, as well as interventions in the current educational framework to promote AI-related competencies in university curricula. However, the regulation of these literacy and training pathways is delegated to governmental decrees, which are to be adopted within one year from the entry into force of the law. Furthermore, the bill does not establish any deadline for the actual implementation of the AI literacy programs. In short, the way planned by the *Law on AI* seems to be antithetical to the one chosen by the European legislator in the AI Act.

A further point of divergence between Art. 7, par. 3, of the *Law on AI* and the AI Act has been highlighted by the European Commission in a detailed opinion on the draft presented by the Italian Government and, later, approved (Opinion C(2024) 7814 of 20 November 2024). The remark focuses on the excessive breadth of the informational obligation that the original version of Art. 7, par. 3, imposes on physicians, who would have been required to inform patients of the "use of artificial intelligence technologies," the "diagnostic and therapeutic benefits" derived from such technologies, and the "decision-making logic" of the system.

In particular, the EU Commission outlines that the Italian legislator seeks to expand medical communication beyond what is required under the AI Act, limited to the use of AI in the provision of healthcare services. Because of this criticism, the Senate has amended the third paragraph of Art. 7 of the bill, so that the final version now only states that the patient has the right to be informed about the AI technologies involved in the medical treatment.

It is also worth emphasising that, by its opinion on the Italian *bill*, the EU Commission has indirectly provided an authentic interpretation of the AI Act's provisions concerning informational duties and the use of AI systems in healthcare. On the basis of the AI Act, healthcare professionals are under a duty to inform patients that the diagnosis or therapy being proposed involves the use of AI technology.

5 Concluding Remarks

The AI Act and the Italian *Law on AI* impose a duty on the doctors to inform their patients about the AI systems involved in medical treatment but do not require a detailed description of this technology and its functioning.

The imposition of a peremptory obligation raises some doubts. First, for the reasons explained above (Sect. 2), a more desirable approach would be the adoption of a flexible rule that allows physicians to calibrate the amount and nature of information disclosed based on the specific circumstances and individual characteristics of each patient. Furthermore, it must be considered that involving the patient in the decision to use AI in diagnosis or therapy risks evolving into recognition of the patient's right to demand that the medical treatment be carried out exclusively by human professionals. However, such an outcome would be in contrast with Art. 1 of Law No. 219/2017, where informed consent is conceived as a point of balance between the patient's decisional autonomy and the physician's professional discretion.

By contrast, the normative choice not to impose on physicians the obligation to provide detailed explanations of the AI systems employed warrants approval, as it appropriately respects the limits of their technical expertise and avoids unnecessary informational burdens.

Moreover, if the law were to oblige physicians to provide a precise explanation of the decision-making logic underlying the AI system employed in treatment, the medical sector would be limited to using only those AI applications that are fully transparent. Such a restriction would ultimately be detrimental to healthcare. Indeed, many AI experts argue that increasing the intelligibility of a system often entails a decrease in its accuracy. This may well explain why, in the AI Act, where both aspects are equally valued, transparency is not mandated to the extent necessary to ensure that the system's decision-making logic is comprehensible to any person (including, in medical contexts, the patient), but only to the degree necessary to enable the person interacting with the AI system (in this case, healthcare professionals) to use it appropriately.

Finally, the informational obligation concerning AI and its underlying decision-making logic could, in certain cases, lead physicians to refrain from using a technology that would otherwise be beneficial to the patient's treatment. Such a risk is well illustrated by the facts that led to a recent judgement of the Italian Supreme Court (Cass. 19 April 2024, no. 22888). Lacking the necessary language skills to explain the tetanus vaccination to a foreign patient, the physician opted not to administer it. Such a decision resulted in the onset of the disease. This case demonstrates that imposing informational duties which the physician is unable to fulfil may ultimately reduce the therapeutic opportunities available to the patient. Such an outcome reflects a new form of defensive medicine, prompted by the fear of incurring liability for violating the requirements of informed consent.

In my view, then, the limits of human knowledge suggest that the physician's informational obligations should be kept within reasonable bounds. However, starting from the same concern, one might propose a different solution. That is, one might consider delegating to a conversational AI system the task of illustrating to the patient every detail of the available treatments and guiding them through the related decision-making process. Such a technology has already been developed and has been named "Consent-GPT".

However, the proposal to delegate the task of informing patients to an AI system seems to be at odds with the core of the considerations developed in this chapter, namely, that self-determination cannot be conceived as a univocal and absolute value. When considering Consent-GPT, the rationales underlying self-determination diverge: on the one hand, they support the potential of an AI system to provide patients with comprehensive information; on the other hand, they raise concerns about biases and misinformation such a system might convey. Moreover, it must be remembered that, as Art. 1 of Law no. 219/2017 clearly states, informed consent is based not only on the patient's decisional autonomy, but also on the trust placed in the physician and on the physician's competence and responsibility. In other words, informed consent cannot be reduced to a mere exchange of information or a procedural formality. It necessarily involves elements that are intrinsically human, such as trust, empathy, interpretive judgement, and the physician's ability to tailor communication to the patient's individual needs and circumstances. These dimensions are not replicable by even the most advanced artificial systems, and their absence would risk compromising the ethical and relational foundations of the consent process.

Bibliography

1. Allen JW, Earp BD, Koplin J, Wilkinson D (2024) Consent-GPT: is it ethical to delegate procedural consent to conversational AI? J Med Ethics 50:77 ff
2. Busnelli FD (2011) Problemi giuridici di fine vita tra natura e artificio. Riv Diritto Civ 161 ff
3. Calderai V (2015) Consenso informato. Enciclopedia del diritto, Annali VIII, pp 225–263
4. Carminati A (2018) Libertà di cura e autonomia del medico. Profili costituzionali. Cacucci, Bari

5. Chieffi L (2019) Il diritto all'autodeterminazione terapeutica. Origine ed evoluzione di un valore costituzionale. Giappichelli, Torino
6. Cohen G (2020) Informed consent and medical artificial intelligence: what to tell to the patient. Georget Law J 108:1432 ff
7. Corradi S (2024) Comprendere la vulnerabilità. Pluralismo ontologico e sistemi di intelligenza artificiale nel diritto. BioLaw J Special Issue:5 ff
8. Daniele V (2022) AI e consenso informato del paziente: quando è possibile, le questioni da risolvere. www.agendadigitale.eu. Accessed 21 July 2022
9. De Menech C (2022) Intelligenza artificiale e autodeterminazione in materia sanitaria. BioLaw J 1:181 ff
10. Foglia M (2018) Consenso e cura. La solidarietà nel rapporto terapeutico. Giappichelli, Torino
11. Morana D, Balduzzi T, Morganti F (2022) La salute "intelligente": eHealth, consenso informato e principio di non-discriminazione 127 ff. www.federalismi.it
12. Santosuosso A, Tosco L (2020) Forum: law and artificial intelligence. BioLaw J, Special Issue:505 ff
13. Nicolussi A (2013) Testamento biologico e problemi del fine-vita: verso un bilanciamento di valori o un nuovo dogma della volontà? Eur Dirit Priv:457 ff
14. Razzano G (2019) La legge n. 219/2017 su consenso informato e DAT fra libertà di cura e rischio di innesti eutanasici. Giappichelli, Torino
15. Rossi E (2011) Profili giuridici del consenso informato: i fondamenti costituzionali e gli ambiti di applicazione. Rivista AIC 4:1 ff
16. Tozzi AE, Cinelli G (2021) Informed consent and artificial intelligence applied to RCT and Covid-19. BioLaw J Special Issue:97 ff
17. Zatti P (2008) Rapporto medico-paziente e «integrità» della persona. In: Nuova giurisprudenza civile commentata Pt. 2:403 ff

Chapter 12
Oncological Oblivion

Salvatore Orlando

1 The Prohibitions on Personal Data Processing Laid Down by Italian Law No. 193/2023

The personal data, considered by Italian Law 7 December 2023, No. 193 (Provisions for the prevention of discrimination and the protection of the rights persons who have been affected by oncological diseases) consist of health data relevant to oncological diseases whose active medical treatment has been completed without recurrences for at least 10 years, or for at least 5 years in case the disease first appeared when the patient was younger than 21 years of age (Art. 2, 3, and 4). For certain specific oncological pathologies, the above-mentioned 10- and 5-year terms are reduced (on account of scientific evidence of different average periods of recovery), as decided upon and formalised by ad hoc procedures and documents, and subject to periodic reviews (Art. 5, par. 2).

Art. 2 of Law 193/2023 prohibits the collection and in any case the processing of any such personal data relevant to a contracting party for the purposes of determining the terms and conditions of any contract whatsoever, even if entered between non-professional parties.

Art. 3 of Law 193/2023 prohibits the collection and processing of the same personal data relevant to prospective adoptive parents in child adoption procedures for the purposes of making by the competent authorities of any decisions on their eligibility as adoptive parents.

Art. 4 of Law 193/2023 prohibits the collection of the same personal data for the purposes of any recruiting or other selection procedures, whether public or private,

S. Orlando (✉)
Sapienza University of Rome—JODI (Juridical Observatory on Digital Innovation), Rome, Italy
e-mail: salvatore.orlando@uniroma1.it

A. Bernes, S. Thobani (eds.), *Digitalisation in Health Care between New Technologies, Data and Research*, Services and Business Process Reengineering, https://doi.org/10.1007/978-981-95-6982-3_12

even in case the procedure in question contemplates the assessment of the health requirements of the candidates.

2 The Reason for the Prohibitions

The reason for the various prohibitions laid down by Law 193/2023 essentially lies, in each case, in the intention to counter discrimination against persons who have recovered from oncological diseases. They are anti-discrimination prohibitions. Therefore, although Art. 1(1) of Law 193/2023 quotes a number of other provisions of primary law, as well as a communication by the European Commission of 2021 titled *Europe's Beating Cancer Plan,*[1] the primary law sources to be looked at for capturing the *ratio legis* of Law 193/2023 are Art. 21 of the Charter of Fundamental Rights of the European Union (CFREU) and Art. 3 of the Italian Constitution, setting forth the general prohibition on discrimination.

This rationale is precisely reflected in the title of Law 193/2023: Provisions for preventing discrimination and for protecting the rights of persons who have been affected by oncological diseases.

The concept of "specification" is useful to understand precisely the relation between Law 193/2023 and the above-mentioned provisions of primary law: the prohibitions provided for by Artt. 2, 3, and 4 of Law 193/2023 are *specifications* of the general prohibition on discrimination stated in Artt. 21 CFREU and 3 of the Italian Constitution. Namely, Artt. 2, 3, and 4 of Law 193/2023 *make the general prohibition on discrimination specific, with specific reference to* the so-called cancer survivors, by prohibiting the discrimination against people having a certain health history which resulted in the recovery from an oncological disease (the so-called cancer survivors) compared to the generality of other contracting parties, applicants, and candidates, in connection, respectively, with (1) any contractual relationships; (2) any child adoption procedures, and (3) any recruiting or other selective procedures, whether public or private, including those procedures contemplating the assessment of health conditions of the relevant candidates.

It is important to underline that there is a medical or scientific ground for the *legal notion* of cancer survivors understood by the Italian legislator. On the basis of medical and scientific data, the Italian legislator *understands* that cancer survivors are—and therefore provides that as a matter of Italian law they "shall be"—those patients that have a certain medical history, namely those patients that have lived without recessions for a number of years after the end of the active medical treatment of the disease. Broadly comparable legal notions of cancer survivors (cancer-free persons) are taken into account by the legislators of other European countries and by the European Parliament (**EP**).

[1] COM(2021) 44 final of 3 February 2021.

Similarly to what provided for by the laws of other European countries (France, Belgium, Luxembourg, The Netherlands, Romania, Spain, UK) and in line with what requested by the EP in point 125 of its resolution *Strengthening Europe in the fight against cancer* of 16 February 2022,[2] Law 193/2023 retains that cancer survivors are those patients that have survived without recurrences for more than 10 years after the end of an active medical treatment, or 5 years if they had their cancer diagnosis before the age of 21. In this latter respect, the notion of "young" cancer survivors retained by Law 193/2023 is different and wider than that understood by the EP in the above-mentioned resolution, in which the relevant age of reference is 18 years old.

Moreover, Law 193/2023 expressly protects cancer survivors against discrimination well beyond their quality as consumers in the financial sector. In fact, as mentioned, cancer survivors are protected by Law 193/2023 against discrimination in their quality as contracting parties in any contractual relationships, as well as in their quality as applicants in child adoption procedures, and in their quality as candidates in any recruiting and other selective procedures.

The rationale of Law 193/2023 brings about some further reflections.

Despite some contrary opinions, Law 193/2023 cannot be interpreted so as to imply that survivors of serious diseases other than cancer may be discriminated against as a matter of Italian or Union law, in the absence of an ad hoc normative as that set forth by Law 193/2023. Least of all, it is correct to maintain that Law 193/2023 is contrary to the Italian Constitution, for being itself discriminatory, in the part it does not contain the same or similar prohibitions for protecting survivors to other serious diseases.

Discrimination is always unlawful. Law 193/2023 simply testifies a broad scientific consensus on the concept of "cancer survivor" and was driven by the urgency to address this matter on account of the seriousness and wide diffusion of cancer pathologies. For the same reasons, laws similar to Law 193/2023 (although not

---

[2] Strengthening Europe in the fight against cancer, European Parliament resolution of 16 February 2022 on strengthening Europe in the fight against cancer—towards a comprehensive and coordinated strategy, P9_TA(2022)0038, point 125: "[...] insurers and banks should not take into account the medical history of people who have been affected by cancer; calls for national legislation to ensure that cancer survivors are not discriminated against compared to other consumers; notes the Commission's intention to engage with businesses to develop a code of conduct to ensure that developments in cancer treatments and their improved effectiveness are reflected in the business practices of financial service providers; supports, in parallel, the promotion of advances made in France, Belgium, Luxembourg and the Netherlands, where cancer survivors enjoy the 'right to be forgotten'; requests that by 2025, at the latest, all Member States should guarantee the right to be forgotten to all European patients 10 years after the end of their treatment, and up to 5 years after the end of treatment for patients whose diagnosis was made before the age of 18; calls for the introduction of common standards for the right to be forgotten under the relevant provisions on consumer protection policy of the Treaty on the Functioning of the European Union, in order to remedy the fragmented national practices in the area of creditworthiness assessment and ensure equal access to credit for cancer survivors; calls for embedding the right to be forgotten for cancer survivors into relevant EU legislation to prevent discrimination and improve cancer survivors' access to financial services".

perfectly identical) have been adopted by a number of other countries and advocated, as said, by the EP.

Also with respect to other serious diseases (such as hepatitis C and HIV), Italian law (Art. 21 of the Italian Constitution) and Union law (Art. 21 CFREU) certainly shall be interpreted and applied in the sense of concluding that it is prohibited to discriminate against people that are cured of those diseases. In other cases—where there are no legal notions of healing, as precisely disposed by Law 193/2023—the occurrence of discriminatory practices can *and shall* be assessed on a case- by-case basis. The relevant requirements, in particular, in terms of recovery periods, need to be specified by case law.

By specifying the general prohibition on discrimination with specific reference to the discrimination against cancer-free persons, the Italian legislator, with Law 193/2023, has removed the doubts and uncertainties which inevitably surround the assessment of the discriminatory nature of the conduct attracting scrutiny of this kind in connection with the oncological class of diseases. But an anti-discrimination scrutiny cannot be limited to cancer survivors. Any such conclusion would be contrary to the general prohibition on discrimination set out in primary law sources, as recalled above (Art. 21 CFREU and Art. 3 of the Italian Constitution).

The above interpretation is confirmed by the provisions on secondary use contained in the recently approved Regulation (EU) 2025/327 on European Health Data Space (EHDS Regulation), whereby not only countering discrimination is one of the tasks each digital health authority shall be entrusted with (Art. 19(2)(h)), but also the following purposes for secondary uses are expressly prohibited, resulting in a prohibition of the correspondent uses:

"[…] taking decisions in relation to a natural person or a group of natural persons in relation to job offers, offering less favourable terms in the provision of goods or services, including exclusion of such persons or groups from the benefit of an insurance or credit contract, the modification of their contributions and insurance premiums or conditions of loans, or taking any other decisions in relation to a natural person or a group of natural persons *which result in discriminating against them on the basis of the health data obtained* […]" (Art. 54(1)(b)).

As it is made clear in the EHDS regulation, an assessment of the kind required by this important provision certainly is not confined to discrimination against cancer survivors and, in the absence of specific law provisions setting requirements and notions such as those provided by Law 193/2023 for cancer diseases, will have to be made on a case-by-case basis.

Two final remarks on contract law: Firstly, it appears correct to observe that companies do not have an economic interest (in itself) to discriminate against cancer survivors, being it true, on the contrary, that—in any truly competitive market and in the absence of cartels or other anticompetitive arrangements—companies would normally find it convenient to seek and offer to cancer survivors the same conditions applied to the generality of the other clients in order to acquire those clients *provided that they were satisfied on their quality as cancer-free persons*. Therefore, Law 193/2023 simply provides certain minimum requirements that shall be complied with in any contractual dealings, while, of course, nothing prevents companies to compete on the basis of their possible reliance on shorter recovery periods than those taken into account by Law 193/2023.

Secondly, as a matter of Italian contract law, it appears correct to maintain that the same regime provided by Art. 2(6) of Law 193/2023 with respect to the discrimination against cancer survivors shall apply for the discrimination against *survivors of any other serious disease*, i.e. the nullity of the contractual clauses that have been determined as a result of the discrimination and the replacement of the invalid clauses, if necessary, with clauses reflecting the terms and conditions applied to the generality of the other clients.

Two final remarks on the expressions "oncological oblivion" and "right to be forgotten".

Once the prohibitions laid down by Artt. 2, 3, and 4 of Law 193/2023 and their reasons are correctly understood, the definition of "right to oncological oblivion" contained in Art. 1(2) of Law 193/2023 appears either redundant or misleading: "the right of the persons recovered from an oncological pathology to not provide information and to not be made subject to investigations about their prior pathological condition in the cases provided by the present law".

In fact, on one side, the word "oblivion" and the expression «right to be forgotten» do not adequately convey the idea that Law 193/2023 is an anti-discrimination law. On the other side, the entire definition appears inconsistent with the legal regime effectively designed by Law 193/2023, consisting, as noted, in a number of prohibitions on the collection and processing of certain personal data for certain purposes.

And effectively, the notion of a "right not to provide certain information" is per se useless if there is no clarity on the consequences of the voluntary provision of the same information, if any, while the notion of a "right to not be made subject to certain investigations" adds nothing (in terms of legal content) to the corresponding prohibition.

Therefore, the only sensible question that one may ask in interpreting this provision is "*what happens if* the personal information on past oncological disease, as precisely considered by Law 193/2023, is *voluntarily given* for any of the processing purposes that are under the prohibitions set by the same law"?

We shall address this question in the next paragraph.

3 The Mandatory Character of the Prohibitions and the Invalidity Pursuant to the GDPR of any Consent Given by the Data Subject for the Processing Purposes Prohibited by Italian Law 193/2023

The mandatory character of the prohibitions laid down by Law 193/2023 derives from their anti-discrimination nature, and, more precisely, from their being specifications of the general prohibition on discrimination set out in primary sources (the CFREU and the Italian Constitution), as illustrated in Sect. 2 above.

With specific regard to the prohibitions relevant to contracts, contained in Art. 2 of Law 193/2023, their mandatory character is confirmed by the provision of Art. 2(6) of Law 193/2023, dictating the nullity of the contractual clauses that have been determined in contrast with the principles of Art. 2(1) in case of violation of the provisions contained in Art. 2, paragraphs from (1) to (5) of Law 193/2023,[3] i.e. as a result of a discriminatory conduct carried out against a cancer survivor.

The violation of the provisions of Art. 2, paragraphs from (1) to (5) of Law 193/2023 amounts to a *typical discriminatory conduct*, designed, as said, by the Italian legislator through "specific" law provisions, in the sense illustrated in paragraph 2 above.

Although Law 193/2023 does not explicitly address the question, it appears correct to maintain that the nullity provided by Art. 2(6) of Law 193/2023 cannot be avoided by a voluntary supply of the relevant information by the cancer survivor and/or by an explicit consent given by the cancer survivor to the processing of the same information for the purpose of determining contractual clauses. In fact, as mentioned, Law 193/2023 provides that this is an illegitimate purpose as the relevant conduct typically amounts to discriminatory conduct against cancer survivors.

Art. 2(6) of Law 193/2023 also provides that the nullity may be assessed by the competent Judge ex officio (i.e. even in case the cancer survivor has not filed or has

[3] "1. For the purposes of entering into or renewing contracts relevant to banking, financial, investment or insurance services, as well as in the context of the entering of any other types of contract, even if exclusively between individuals, whenever, at the time of the conclusion of the contract or at a later stage, the information are capable to affect the contractual terms and conditions, it is prohibited to request information relevant to the health conditions of the contracting party concerning oncological pathologies that previously affected the contracting party and whose active treatment has ended without episodes of relapse for more than 10 years at the date of the request. This period is reduced by an half in case the pathology appeared before the 21st year of age. The information under this paragraph cannot be collected neither from sources other than the contracting party, and in any case, where already available to the professional or the intermediary, cannot be used for determining the contractual conditions.

2. In all phases of access to banking, financial, investment or insurance services, including during the negotiation, the conclusion or the renewal of contracts, banks, credit institutions, insurance companies and financial and insurance intermediaries shall provide the counterparty with adequate information on the right under paragraph 1, of which express mention shall be made in the standard forms and models prepared and used for the purposes of the conclusion and the renewal of the said contracts.

3. In the cases contemplated under paragraphs 1 and 2 above, it is prohibited to apply to the counterparty limits, costs, and burdens in excess or different regimes compared to those provided for the generality of the contractual counterparties according to the applicable laws and regulation.

4. In the cases contemplated under paragraph1 above, banks, credit institutions, insurance companies and financial and insurance intermediaries shall not request to carry out medical inspections or clinical analyses for the conclusion of the contracts mentioned in the same paragraph.

5. In case the information mentioned in paragraph 1 above have been provided before the completion of the term mentioned under the same paragraph, they cannot be used afterward for the purposes of evaluating the risk of the transaction or the creditworthiness of the contracting party. To this extent, the contracting party timely sends to the bank, or credit institution, or insurance company or financial or insurance intermediary, via registered letter or certified email, the certification released in accordance with the provisions of the decree provided by article 5, paragraph 1. Within 30 days from the receipt of the said certification, the professionals mentioned above in possession of the information under paragraph 1 of the present article shall procure their cancellation".

not filed timely any such request) and may only operate so as to benefit the cancer survivor and not also her/his contract counterparty. This provision—which is very common in consumer law (so-called *protective nullity*)—is exclusively and precisely intended to avoid opportunistic behaviours on the part of the party that has caused the invalidity of the contract, and cannot be interpreted for supporting the view that a consent given by the cancer survivor to the processing of her/his personal data for those specific purposes that are prohibited by Law 193/2023 is capable of avoiding the nullity in question.

It also follows from the mandatory character of the prohibitions laid down by Law 193/2023 that if the cancer survivor gives her/his consent to the processing of the personal data that are under the prohibitions of Law 193/2023 for the purposes that are prohibited by Law 193/2023, the processing of those personal data shall be deemed unlawful not only as a matter of Law 193/2023 (with the consequences provided therein) but also as a matter of the GDPR, with the consequences provided by the GDPR.

In this respect, the provision of Art. 5(1)(b) GDPR shall certainly be applied and needs to be coordinated with that of Art. 6(1)(a) GDPR.

Art. 5(1)(b) GDPR provides that data shall be collected and processed for *legitimate purposes*.

The coordination between the two provisions shall be made, maintaining that Art. 5(1)(b) GDPR, contemplating and imposing a legitimacy test on the specific purposes of the processing of personal data, must necessarily be coupled with that of Art. 6(1)(a) GDPR, so as to conclude that when the data subject gives consent to the processing "for one or more specific purposes", those purposes shall be "legitimate".

As a consequence, any consent to processing activities for purposes that are prohibited by Law 193/2023 shall be deemed invalid pursuant to the GDPR, with the consequences attached to the unlawful processing of personal data as provided for by the GDPR.

As I will illustrate in the next paragraph, the above interpretation of Law 193/2023 is consistent with an important feature of contemporary EU data law.

4 The Many Direct and Indirect Prohibitions on the Processing of Certain Personal Data for Certain Purposes Set Out in Contemporary Sources of Union and National Law and the "Substantive" Test of Lawfulness of Personal Data Processing Under the GDPR

With the advent of the data industry and the spread of AI systems—and the consequent passage from the "information society" to the "data-driven society"—it is necessary to consolidate the view that, as long as the interpretation and application of the GDPR is concerned, the processing of personal data shall pass a "substantive" test of lawfulness aimed at assessing the observance or non-violation of mandatory provisions of Union and national law that directly or indirectly provide prohibitions on the processing of certain personal data for certain purposes. Such a test shall be carried out in relation to any of the conditions or bases requested by the GDPR for the lawful processing of personal data.

Although not clearly spelt out, this actually is an implicit requirement by the GDPR, since, also on the basis of Art. 5(1)(b) of the GDPR, which, as noted, makes clear that personal data shall be collected and processed for legitimate purposes:

(a) Consent by the data subject to the processing of her/his personal data for one or more specific purposes shall be read as necessarily referring to *legitimate* purposes
(b) Performance of a contract shall necessarily be read as performance of a *legitimate* contract

each and all of the conditions sub letters (c), (d), and (e) of Art. 6(1) GDPR—i.e. (c) compliance with a legal obligation, (d) protecting vital interests, and (e) performance of a task carried out in the public interest or in the exercise of official authority vested in the controller— by definition shall be intended to refer to *legitimate* purposes and activities; and, finally (f) legitimate interests, too, cannot, by definition, imply illegitimate purposes or activities.

A number of sources of contemporary EU data law present mandatory provisions containing either direct or indirect prohibitions on processing certain data for certain purposes.

As regards direct prohibitions, we can cite the Directive (EU) 2024/2831 on improving working conditions in platform work, the Regulation (EU) 2022/2065, also known as the Digital Services Act (DSA), the Regulation (EU) 2024/900 on the transparency and targeting of political advertising, and the EHDS Regulation.

As regards indirect prohibitions, we can cite the Regulation (EU) 2024/1689 on artificial intelligence (AI Act).

Coming very briefly to each source: pursuant to Art. 7 of the directive on online platform workers, digital labour platforms (as defined therein) are prohibited from processing by means of automated decision-making or monitoring systems (as defined therein): (a) personal data relating to the emotional or psychological state of the person performing platform work; (b) personal data relating to private conversations; (c) personal data where the person performing platform work is not performing platform work or is not offering to do so; (d) personal data to provide for the exercise of fundamental rights, including the right of association, the right to collective bargaining and collective action, or the right to information and consultation, as defined in the Charter of Fundamental Rights of the European Union; (e) personal data to infer a person's racial or ethnic origin, migrant status, political opinions, religious or philosophical beliefs, disability, state of health, including chronic diseases or HIV status, emotional or psychological state, membership of a trade union, sex life or sexual orientation; (f) biometric data, as defined in the GDPR, of a person performing platform work to establish his or her identity by comparing it with the biometric data of persons stored in a database.

Prohibitions on processing certain personal data (those under Art. 9(1) GDPR) for certain marketing purposes are imposed by both the DSa (Art. 26(3)) and the Regulation on political advertising (Art. 18(1)(c)), and the DSA also contains a similar prohibition on processing personal data of minors (Art. 28(2)).

Finally, as mentioned, the EHDS Regulation contains a number of prohibitions on certain secondary uses of health electronic data (Art. 54).

With indirect prohibitions, we make reference to those mandatory rules that do not directly prohibit certain processing activities, but that prohibit certain other activities which necessarily and typically presuppose certain data-processing activities.

The most evident example is that of the prohibitions laid down in Art. 5 of the AI Act on concerning the placing on the market, putting into service, and the use of certain AI systems. Any processing of personal data for the development and use of those systems shall be deemed carried out for an illegitimate purpose, thus qualifying as an unlawful processing pursuant to the GDPR.

But there is no reason to limit the analysis to the provisions of the AI Act, because there are automated processing of personal data, including automated processing of personal data carried out by AI systems, which can be considered unlawful on the basis of other mandatory provisions.

We can think, for example, of online platforms that process personal data for games of chance or prize competitions in violation of mandatory provisions of national laws governing these activities.

Even in such cases, the related processing of personal data will have to be considered unlawful under the GDPR (including, of course, in cases in which the platforms in question make use of artificial intelligence systems).

And in fact, in similar cases we would certainly be in the presence of a violation of the principle expressed by Art. 5(1)(b) GDPR, according to which personal data must be collected for legitimate purposes.

In all these cases, any data subject's consent (pursuant to Art. 6(1) GDPR) or explicit consent (pursuant to Artt. 9(2) or 22(2)(c) GDPR) would be invalid as it would be given for illegitimate purposes and in violation of mandatory provisions of Union or national law.

For all these reasons, Law 193/2023 is perfectly consistent with EU contemporary data law as it provides a number of direct prohibitions on the processing of certain personal data for certain purposes.

The two important issues that need to be addressed in contemporary EU data law, as a consequence of the need for a substantive test on the lawfulness of personal data processing, in the sense outlined above, are: (1) the procurement by the competent authorities of sufficient and adequate technological resources for carrying out the necessary analyses on the automated processing of electronic data and (2) the distribution of competences among the data protection authorities (on one side) and the other administrative and/or judiciary authorities that have the competence to enforce the mandatory provisions prohibiting either directly or indirectly certain processing activities in the various fields of law (on the other side).

In the specific case of Law 193/2023, no such problem of competence exists, since Art. 5(4) of Law 193/2023 has vested the Italian data protection authority with the powers to supervise the enforcement of the Italian law on the so-called oncological oblivion.

Bibliography

1. Campagna M (2024) Il diritto all'oblio oncologico ed il diritto all'oblio nel regolamento privacy dell'UE: assonanze e dissonanze. Nuove leggi civili commentate 5:1163 ff
2. Candido A (2024) Il diritto all'oblio oncologico nel prisma dei diritti della personalità. Nuove leggi civili commentate 5:1146 ff
3. Faccioli M (2025) Le esigenze di tutela delle persone guarite dal cancro e le soluzioni del legislatore italiano. In: Faccioli M (ed) Il diritto all'oblio oncologico. Commentario alla L. 7 dicembre 2023, n. 193. Pacini, Pisa, 1 ff
4. Faccioli M (2025) La disciplina dei contratti con individui titolari del diritto all'oblio oncologico. In: Faccioli M (ed) Il diritto all'oblio oncologico. Commentario alla L. 7 dicembre 2023, n. 193. Pacini, Pisa, 34 ff
5. Faccioli M (2025) Disposizioni transitorie e finali della legge sul diritto all'oblio oncologico. In: Faccioli M (ed) Il diritto all'oblio oncologico. Commentario alla L. 7 dicembre 2023, n. 193. Pacini, Pisa, 81 ff
6. Foglia M (2025) Fondamenti costituzionali e sovranazionali del diritto all'oblio oncologico. In: Faccioli M (ed) Il diritto all'oblio oncologico. Commentario alla L. 7 dicembre 2023, n. 193. Pacini, Pisa, 17 ff
7. Orlando S (2024) Sulla necessità di un controllo di liceità sostanziale per tutte le basi del trattamento dei dati personali. Persona e Mercato 3:815 ff
8. Orlando S (2025) Il regolamento EHDS nel sistema del nuovo diritto europeo dei dati. In: Morace Pinelli A (ed) Il regolamento EHDS. Commentario. Pacini, Pisa, forthcoming
9. Orlando S (2025) Reflections upon 'the privacy fallacy' by Ignacio Cofone. Eur J Privacy Law Technol, forthcoming
10. Paladini M (2024) Il diritto all'oblio oncologico: obblighi e divieti contrattuali. Nuove leggi civili commentate 5:1063 ff
11. Peruzzi M (2025) Oblio oncologico e tutela della persona che lavora. In: Faccioli M (ed) Il diritto all'oblio oncologico. Commentario alla L. 7 dicembre 2023, n. 193. Pacini, Pisa, p 71 ff
12. Renda A (2024) Il diritto all'oblio oncologico e l'adozione. Nuove leggi civili commentate 5:1085 ff
13. Vizzoni L (2025) L'adozione da parte del cancer survivor fra diritto all'oblio oncologico e tutela dell'interesse del minore. In: Faccioli M. (ed.) Il diritto all'oblio oncologico. Commentario alla L. 7 dicembre 2023, n. 193. Pacini, Pisa, 53 ff

Chapter 13
Clinical Trials, Scientific Research, and Liability

Massimo Foglia

1 Introduction

The subject of this reflection—liability in scientific research and clinical trials—requires a twofold framing: on the one hand, the discipline of scientific research and its prerequisites (in particular, informed consent and the processing of personal data); on the other hand, the discipline of clinical trials (e.g. in the field of pharmacology), with its regulatory framework and liability models.

Here we confine ourselves to some transversal considerations, proposed in a problematic key, and which find a point of intersection in the use of artificial intelligence (AI) in biomedical research.

With reference to emerging legal issues, the question was raised, for instance, who was liable in the event of an error in the use of an AI system during experimentation? And in this regard, it was discussed whether it was necessary to redefine the traditional categories of fault and strict liability. Or it was observed how the use of AI requires models of informed consent that take into account the evolution of algorithms and potential changes in data processing (the concept of so-called dynamic informed consent was also alluded to here). And again, attention has been drawn to the fact that the use of AI may exacerbate inequalities in access to clinical trials, especially in developing countries.

These are just a few examples. It is appropriate, as a preliminary step, to provide some contextual background in order to properly frame the discussion concerning the potential of AI technologies and their applications in the fields of scientific research and clinical trials.

M. Foglia (✉)
University of Bergamo, Bergamo, Italy
e-mail: massimo.foglia@unibg.it

A. Bernes, S. Thobani (eds.), *Digitalisation in Health Care between New Technologies, Data and Research*, Services and Business Process Reengineering, https://doi.org/10.1007/978-981-95-6982-3_13

2 Artificial Intelligence as Tool and Object of Research

Today, AI is used both as a support tool for scientific activities and as the object of experimentation itself. In the first case, it contributes to the organisation and processing of clinical and biological data; in the second, it is evaluated to verify its predictive and therapeutic potential, also for regulatory purposes.

If we think of AI as a tool, we see that by using advanced techniques such as machine learning and deep learning, AI speeds up data processing, reducing time and costs in the discovery of new drugs; it also facilitates the analysis of large amounts of chemical, biological, and clinical data, identifying promising molecules and reducing toxicity and side effects; and it supports the selection of participants for clinical trials and the optimisation of therapies already on the market, identifying new ways of use and improving therapeutic benefits for patients.

As pointed out in the European Medicines Agency (EMA) *Reflection Paper on the use of AI in the medicinal product lifecycle* (9 September 2024),[1] artificial intelligence is at every stage of the medicinal product lifecycle: from pre-clinical research to the selection of clinical trial participants and from manufacturing to post-marketing surveillance. The "algorithmic" nature of the processes, however, makes the attribution of responsibility opaque, complicating the regulatory framework. The complexity of the computational model can make it difficult to identify the aetiological moment of the error and the liable party.

If, on the other hand, we imagine AI as an object of study, we observe that AI is studied to assess its diagnostic, prognostic, and therapeutic efficacy; and it requires in-depth analyses of the quality of results, cost-effectiveness, and management of clinical data.

In both functions, AI aims to improve scientific knowledge and therapeutic outcomes, contributing to the well-being of people and society.

3 The EU AI Act and Regulatory Gaps

However, there are also inherent risks in the development and use of this specific technology, in terms of opacity, discrimination, misuse of clinical data, or overreliance on intelligent systems. And so ensuring that these risks are minimised must be a cornerstone in the use of AI in the context of medical research, to ensure effective protection of people's rights within this dimension.

From this perspective, it would therefore seem appropriate to question and reflect on what rules and guarantees should apply in cases where AI becomes relevant in medical research, both as a tool and as the object of this activity, in order to provide

[1] www.ema.europa.eu/en/documents/scientific-guideline/reflection-paper-use-artificial-intelligence-ai-medicinal-product-lifecycle_en.

researchers (and people in general) with greater certainty as to the possibilities of using intelligent systems and the consequences that may ensue.

Now, I would like to focus on the most recent European regulation on artificial intelligence (Regulation (EU) 2024/1689, also known as AI Act). Because the AI Act introduced a regulatory framework that regulates scientific research and clinical trials with AI systems in different ways, placing particular emphasis on risk-based management.

With specific regard to scientific research, the regulation provides an exemption for AI systems developed and used exclusively for scientific research or development purposes, provided they are not intended to be placed on the market or put into service for commercial purposes. This principle is enshrined in Art. 2, par. 6 and 8, with the aim of not hindering innovation and respecting scientific freedom.

But then there are limitations to the exemption. The exemption does not apply to tests under real conditions or to AI systems subsequently placed on the market. The regulation emphasises that research activities must comply with EU ethical and professional regulations, as clarified in Recital 25 and Recital 142.

We know that the regulation adopts a model that classifies AI systems according to their level of risk (high, limited, minimal). And for low-risk systems used in scientific research, the AI Act provides for minimum obligations such as transparency (Art. 50) and voluntary codes of conduct (Art. 95).

With regard to clinical trials, however, we must distinguish between AI as a medical research tool and AI as a research object.

In the former case, the use of AI to improve processes such as data analysis, drug discovery, and selection of participants in clinical trials does fall within the framework of the AI Act, which, however, does not classify these applications as high risk, with some exceptions (e.g. if they involve medical devices or triage systems, as stated in Annex III). Whereas when AI is the subject of clinical research, the AI Act requires compliance with the applicable regulations for high-risk systems, including requirements for risk management, transparency, human oversight, and technical documentation (Chap. 3, Sect. 2). However, these regulations may not be sufficient to mitigate risks such as data bias or opacity in advanced models.

4 EMA Guidance and Final Considerations

Thus, there are some criticalities noted by observers. A first critical issue concerns a lack of ethical oversight. The AI Act does not provide for a mandatory ethics committee to supervise clinical research with AI, creating a possible gap in the protection of fundamental rights and research integrity. Secondly, there could be a problem of fairness for public bodies. The uniform application of rules to public and private entities could penalise public research, which is limited by lower economic resources than those available to the private sector. Finally, a need for regulatory coordination was noted. The complexity of the legal landscape would require harmonisation between the AI Act and other European regulations, such as those on data protection and medical devices.

In summary, the AI Act is an important step towards a unified regulation of scientific and clinical research with AI, but it presents challenges that will require further regulatory and interpretative action.

Lastly, I would like to make a reference to a recent document, which I think is worth mentioning because—although it has no regulatory value—it is a useful reference point with regard to the clinical testing of medicines. This is the abovementioned Reflection Paper on the use of AI in the medicinal product lifecycle presented on 9 September 2024 by the EMA, in which important considerations are made on the integration of AI systems within the drug lifecycle and in which the foundations are laid for future publications on the subject of AI.

In the wake of the Discussion Paper presented by the US Food and Drug Administration on the same topic in May 2023, the Reflection Paper contains the EMA's considerations on the use of AI to "support the safe and effective development, production and use of [...] drugs".

In particular, the Reflection Paper identifies the areas of use of AI in the drug lifecycle where the EMA itself or national regulatory authorities have the power to intervene, highlighting critical issues and possible corrective measures. As far as pharmaceutical research is concerned, the risk arising from the use of AI normally falls on the sponsor and particular caution is recommended in cases where the results produced by the AI contribute substantially to the formation of the drug authorisation dossier submitted to the regulatory authorities.

From this point of view, I would just like to point out that the issue of the use of AI in drug trials—and of the possible consequent liability arising from the use of this technology—is part of a case in which a plurality of subjects are involved on different levels the *promoter* of the trial, i.e. the pharmaceutical company that produces the experimental drug; the *experimental centre*, i.e. the hospital company that is responsible for administering the treatment to the patients included in the project; the *investigating doctors*, who are usually auxiliaries of the hospital company itself and interact directly with the patients recruited, both in the phase of selecting the recipients of the experimental treatment and in that of administering the therapy; and of course the *subject*, i.e. the patient, who adheres, by giving his consent, to the trial (see Art. 2 of Legislative Decree No. 211 of 24 June 2003, entitled "Implementation of Directive 2001/20/EC on the implementation of good clinical practice in the conduct of clinical trials on medicinal products for clinical use").

From the point of view of the allocation of responsibilities, even before the advent of AI, jurisprudence was called upon to resolve this "complicated juggling of legal relations"—to use an expression by Rosario Nicolò (*L'adempimento dell'obbligo altrui*, Milan, 1936, 11). And so it is in this scenario that the new implications arising from the use of AI must also be addressed.

Returning to the EMA Reflection Paper and the critical issues raised on the areas of use of AI, I would also like to point out the one concerning the pre-clinical studies and the product information.

With reference to pre-clinical studies, AI systems should comply with applicable good practices—Good Laboratory Practice (GLP)—aimed at ensuring that pre-clinical studies are organised and conducted according to criteria that promote their safety and quality. And, with regard to product information, AI enables the automation of the drafting of the documentation that must accompany the medicine (e.g. summary of product characteristics, package leaflet). And subsequent verification of the correctness of the contents is recommended.

In this context, EMA sets out the principles that should guide the use of AI in the drug life cycle. The first concerns the responsibility of those involved in the marketing of the medicine, who are responsible for verifying that AI systems are "fit for purpose and in line with the ethical, technical, scientific and regulatory standards described in European legislation, Good Practice standards and current EMA scientific guidelines". Those responsible for marketing the medicine must also adopt a risk-based approach, in which AI risks are assessed according to the specific technology, the stage of the drug's life cycle and the degree of influence exerted by the human component operating the system; and maintain an ongoing dialogue with the regulatory authorities.

The second principle, on the other hand, is a focus on technology: therefore, it is necessary to limit the risks posed by the permeability of AI systems to errors in the data made available to them with: transparency in the selection of data sources and data processing operations; and the creation of a database that is as objective and "cleaned" of biases and errors as possible.

Added to this, of course, are a number of ethical principles, which I will not go into here.

I will only conclude by emphasising that, as the EMA itself has already announced, the Reflection Paper will serve as the basis for further guidelines on the use of AI within the drug life cycle. In fact, the future publication of scientific guidelines on the use of AI in the pharmaceutical field has already been announced, in which the themes and principles set out in the Reflection Paper will be further explored.

It therefore remains to be seen how the current regulatory framework will evolve and, in particular, what policies will be implemented to promote the use of reliable and flexible AI systems also in the pharmaceutical field.

The use of artificial intelligence in clinical trials constitutes a test case for the systemic resilience of civil law. The network of relationships established between promoter, centre, investigator, AI provider and enrolled subject poses the problem of distributed and multilevel liability, which must take into account the principle of accountability and the need for effective protection of the individual.

It is within this framework that the reflection on the relationship between law and science takes place, where standardisation cannot chase technology, but must attempt to govern it without stifling its development.

Bibliography

1. Irti C (2024) Riflessioni sull'impatto delle applicazioni tecnologiche nell'ambito sanitario, tra regole etiche e regole giuridiche, Eur J Privacy Law Technol, 1: 34 ff
2. Massimino F (2000) I contratti di sperimentazione clinica. Contratti, 183 ff
3. Nicolò R (1936) L'adempimento dell'obbligo altrui. Milan, 11

Chapter 14
Artificial Intelligence, Risk Regulation, and Civil Liability: A Legal Analysis of the EU AI Act

Martina D'Onofrio

1 The Artificial Intelligence Act in Europe

The increasing use of artificial intelligence (hereinafter AI) in every sector of human activity has made it necessary to regulate this phenomenon.

In 2024, the so-called Artificial Intelligence Act (henceforth AI Act or Regulation), i.e. a legislative act of the European Union that aims to introduce a harmonised discipline on artificial intelligence at the European level, was adopted. The European Union chose a horizontal regulation, which applies to all areas in which intelligent systems are used, instead of opting for different sectoral regulations.

This is the first European Union regulatory intervention specifically devoted to artificial intelligence, after the European Parliament Resolution of 16 February 2017 with recommendations to the Commission on civil law rules on robotics and the subsequent publication of the White Paper on Artificial Intelligence in February 2020.

The AI Act contains a variety of provisions aimed at preventing potential harm caused by AI systems. The central aim of the Regulation is to ensure the safe use of artificial intelligence and to anticipate the risks that may arise from it.

It is therefore a regulation that attempts to manage the risks arising from the use of AI. On the other hand, it makes no provision for the allocation of liability and remedies in the event of illegal acts performed by intelligent machines. In this respect, a Proposal for a Directive on AI Liability has already been published and will complement the Regulation in the future.

M. D'Onofrio (✉)
University of Milan-Bicocca, Milan, Italy
e-mail: martina.donofrio@unimib.it

A. Bernes, S. Thobani (eds.), *Digitalisation in Health Care between New Technologies, Data and Research*, Services and Business Process Reengineering, https://doi.org/10.1007/978-981-95-6982-3_14

This essay examines the risk management system established by the Regulation and seeks to assess whether, and to what extent, compliance with the obligations under the Regulation excludes the liability of the user of the AI system when it causes damage. For this purpose, it is first necessary to outline the risk classification provided for in the Regulation.

2 The Risk Management System in the AI Act

The structure of the AI Act is entirely based on the management of risks arising from the use of artificial intelligence systems: in fact, the Regulation sets a risk-based approach.

The concept of risk underlying the AI Act is rather traditional and consists of the probability that a hazard will result in loss, injury, or damage.

First of all, the regulation classifies AI systems according to their risk factor, dividing them into four categories: unacceptable, high, limited, and minimal risk.

AI systems are subdivided on the basis of the technology used, with reference to generally identified areas of application (e.g. education, justice, democratic processes, and essential services). However, there are no risk assessments based on concrete application scenarios.

For each of the risk classes, the EU legislator lays down prohibitions, mandatory minimum requirements to be considered in the design and development of AI systems, or transparency obligations or, again, for systems that are less prone to generating risks, simple measures to promote self-regulation. The aim is to set rules that are proportionate to the interests to be protected and the associated risks, with the intention of preventing or mitigating the harmful consequences of AI as efficiently as possible.

To summarise, in Article 5 the AI Act prohibits, with exceptions, devices that produce unacceptable risks; it dedicates the entire Chapter III to the stringent compliance obligations laid down for high-risk systems, while it gradually reduces the obligations for limited and, finally, minimal-risk systems.

The category of tools involving unacceptable risk includes AI systems aimed at psychological manipulation, exploitation of vulnerabilities, biometric categorisation, social scoring, and emotion recognition. For such tools, the AI Act establishes a general prohibition, but provides for some exceptions. For instance, the use of biometric categorisation systems is permitted in certain cases where they intervene in the fight against terrorism.

The category to which the AI Act devotes most provisions, however, is that of high-risk systems, i.e. those that "have a significant harmful impact on the health, safety and fundamental rights of persons", for which a continuous risk management system is envisaged, involving data control, technical documentation, tracking systems, a Fundamental Rights Impact Assessment (FRIA), and the implementation of post-marketing monitoring tools.

Then there are other provisions concerning limited-risk devices (e.g. chatbots), for which mere transparency obligations are envisaged, and minimal-risk devices (e.g. spam filtering mechanisms), for which codes of conduct are optional.

Under this system, as anticipated, the regulatory burdens are distributed proportionally: lesser dangers will require lesser precautions on the part of, for instance, developers and providers of AI systems.

If an AI system meets these requirements and thus adopts the risk mitigation measures required by the regulation, the residual risks associated with each hazard, as well as the overall residual risk, are considered "acceptable".

There are several reasons why the EU legislator decided to have a system involving an ex ante risk assessment.

First, a prognostic and future-oriented view makes it possible to provide sufficiently flexible rules in a constantly changing environment.

Moreover, such an approach makes it possible to effectively protect values and interests that are not always translated into subjective positions recognised by the legal system, as is often the case in the digital sector, as well as to govern the potential hazard arising from dangers that are still partly unknown and whose consequences are difficult to foresee and to quantify precisely.

This does not detract from the fact that the choice made raises some critical issues: first of all, as new inventions are added, it could be complicated to bring them back within the framework already provided by the AI Act; moreover, the current risk classification is drawn up on the basis of current knowledge and use of the systems and may not be able to adapt to any new applications.

3 The Remedial Framework of the AI Act

As already noted, the AI Act provides for compliance obligations that operate ex ante. Nevertheless, it also provides for remedies in the event that these obligations are breached.

First of all, administrative sanctions are provided for operators who violate the obligations set out in the Regulation. The identification of sanctions of a non-monetary nature, which may be associated with or replaced by fines, remains with the Member States, according to principles of effectiveness, proportionality, and deterrence.

The Regulation—unlike other European legal acts, such as the GDPR—does not, on the other hand, expressly provide for ex post compensatory instruments to protect violated subjective legal positions.

For the reasons outlined in the previous paragraph, from an economic analysis of law perspective, it is believed that, in the context of regulating the use of AI, a system that provides for ex ante safeguards is preferable to ex post compensatory protection mechanisms.

Indeed, as has already been argued on the subject of environmental damage, it has been observed that the technical complexity of AI systems would make it very burdensome to meet the burden of proof incumbent on the injured party in compensation proceedings, thus discouraging individual access to ex post forms of compensation protection, especially in systems in which the use of class actions is not yet widespread.

In the field of artificial intelligence, any civil liability remedies would therefore be of a purely contingent and hypothetical nature and would therefore be ineffective and incapable of deterring dangerous conducts of producers and users of AI systems.

It is clear, however, that such an approach leaves open several questions of interpretation. The risk is to create cases where fundamental rights are violated, but the subject is not liable because he or she has correctly complied with the requirements of the Regulation. It is therefore appropriate to question the liability regime to be applied when the rights of individuals who come into contact with intelligent machines are violated.

4 The Management of the So-Called Residual Risk: Liability Under Article 2050 of the Italian Civil Code?

As already noted, the AI Act does not deal with regulating the liability of artificial intelligence, on which, therefore, numerous questions remain open.

In particular, one of the nodal questions arising from the AI Act is that of the compensability of the so-called residual risk, i.e. the risk that remains even after mitigation measures have been taken.

The danger that a regulation such as the AI Act brings with it is that the fulfilment of the risk mitigation measures prescribed by law may, in many cases, constitute a considerable obstacle to the assertion of liability.

Interpreters have long wondered about the provisions applicable in the event of damage resulting from the use of artificial intelligence: indeed, if there is almost unanimity regarding the denial of a subjectification of AI, which would lead to its direct liability, the debate remains heated as to the applicability to the cases in question of the rules set out in Articles 2049 et seq. of the Italian Civil Code, concerning cases of strict or aggravated liability provided for by our system.

In particular, in the event of damage occurring in the context of an activity involving the use of an artificial intelligence system that falls within those classified as "high-risk" by the Regulation, one could hypothesise the applicability of liability pursuant to Article 2050 of the Italian Civil Code for the exercise of a dangerous activity, according to which the exerciser of a dangerous activity is obliged to pay compensation for the damage, if he does not prove that he has adopted all suitable measures to avoid the damage.

The judgment of suitability required by Article 2050 of the Italian Civil Code actually consists of an *ex-ante* assessment of the adequacy of the precautions used to mitigate the risk arising from the dangerous activity. It is, in fact, irrelevant whether such measures later prove to be insufficient in practice to avoid the harmful event.

Indeed, if the judgment were to be carried out a posteriori, suitability would always be denied for the very fact that the means employed were not capable of preventing the occurrence of the harm, so that the only way in which the operator could be exonerated from liability would be to provide proof contrary to the very existence of the harm.

Since the suitability assessment required by Art. 2050 of the Italian Civil Code must also take place ex ante, one might be led to believe that the proof of having taken "appropriate measures to avoid the damage" is satisfied by compliance with all the preventive compliance obligations under the new AI Act. Indeed, it would be possible to think that in such a case, the "appropriate measures" referred to in the letter of the code are typified by the Regulation.

Against this approach, however, two arguments could be raised: one relating to the consistency of the obligations provided for by the Regulation, the other, instead, concerning the interpretation accepted by domestic case law with regard to the release proof granted by Article 2050 of the Italian Civil Code.

In particular, in the first place, with regard to risk mitigation measures, the Regulation provides guidelines that are set at too general and abstract a level to represent the "suitable measures" that should exempt from liability those who use high-risk systems in their business. More technical and specific provisions for individual hazardous activities would be needed in order to be able to consider the burden of proof of liability under the code provision to be discharged.

With regard to the second profile, it is necessary to analyse the reading of the last clause of Article 2050 of the Italian Civil Code that is widespread in living law today.

In this regard, jurisprudence has emphasised that the presumption of liability contemplated by Article 2050 of the Italian Civil Code can only be overcome with particularly rigorous proof, i.e. with the demonstration of having adopted all appropriate measures to avoid the damage. Therefore, negative proof of not having committed any violation of the rules of law or common prudence is not sufficient, but positive proof of having taken every care or measure to prevent the harmful event is required.

If these principles are interpreted in the context of the present case, it is clear that, if the case-law's approach is accepted, it would not be sufficient for the user of a high-risk artificial intelligence system to prove that he has complied with all the provisions laid down by the regulation for such a category of machines.

It seems preferable, therefore, to reject the approach according to which compliance with the provisions of the AI Act would be sufficient to release oneself from liability under Article 2050 of the Italian Civil Code.

On the other hand, if the contrary were to be argued, the result would be that the injured third party would have to bear the burden of the harm arising out of an event occurring in connection with the use of the AI system, provided that the rules of the Regulation had been complied with when the machine was manufactured and used.

Now, the approach just proposed would appear to be in line with the aim of encouraging the development of new AI technologies; however, this outcome is, on closer inspection, very unfair: it would seem more appropriate that risks which cannot be contained by adopting the precautions provided for in the Regulation should be borne by the user for two reasons.

Firstly, it would seem appropriate that the risks arising from the use of AI, which cannot be neutralised by compliance with precautionary measures, should be borne by those who take advantage of it of their own free will, in accordance with the principle *cuius commoda eius et incommoda.*

Moreover, those who produce or use AI systems also have greater control over them than those who merely come into contact with them and have to suffer any damage caused by them.

For these reasons, there seems to be reason to conclude that the injured party in the context of the use of high-risk AI systems is entitled to claim compensation for damages from the user, i.e. the operator of the dangerous activity, if the conditions required by Article 2050 of the Italian Civil Code are met.

However, this does not detract from the fact that when the harmful event is due to a defect in the machine, the user has the right to claim against the manufacturer or other parties (e.g. importer, distributor, deployer, etc.) when the causes of the injury are attributable to them.

5 Concluding Remarks

The analysis of the system outlined by the AI Act highlights a strongly prevention-oriented regulatory framework, based on an ex ante risk management approach.

As noted, this approach, although consistent with the need for flexibility and technological innovation, nevertheless leaves significant questions open in terms of liability. In particular, the treatment of the so-called residual risk today appears to be lacking a complete discipline and there are margins of uncertainty as to the effective protection of the injured party.

While waiting for legislation on the liability of the AI that provides for a specific regulation of the case, Article 2050 of the Italian Civil Code represents an interpretative tool potentially capable of filling this gap, since it is applicable to hazardous activities even when performed in compliance with regulatory obligations. However, its operability requires a strict scrutiny of the appropriateness of the measures taken, which cannot be resolved in mere compliance with the AI Act's compliance obligations.

Therefore, compliance with regulatory requirements, while necessary, cannot be considered sufficient to exclude the user's liability. Such a conclusion would not only be unfair to the injured party but also incompatible with the general principles of the legal system, which require that the risks connected with technological activity be allocated to those who voluntarily undertake it and benefit from it.

It would therefore seem desirable for a supplementary regulatory intervention, which, alongside the preventive regulation contained in the AI Act, would provide a clear framework for civil liability, capable of ensuring effective protection of injured rights and at the same time not discouraging innovation. In the meantime, it remains the task of the interpreter to fill this gap with solutions consistent with the principles of non-contractual liability and with a fair balance between opposing interests.

Bibliography

1. Alpa G (2022) Quale modello normativo per l'intelligenza artificiale? In Buzzelli D, Palazzo M (eds) Intelligenza artificiale e diritti della persona. Pisa, pp 17–38
2. Amidei A (2022) La proposta di Regolamento UE per un 'Artificial Intelligence Act': prime riflessioni sulle ricadute in tema di responsabilità da intelligenza artificiale. Tecnol Diritto, pp 1–34
3. Arnaudo L, Pardolesi R (2023) Ecce robot. Sulla responsabilità dei sistemi adulti di intelligenza artificiale. Danno Resp, pp 409–417
4. Bevivino G (2022) Situazioni giuridiche 'soggettive' e forme di tutela dell'intelligenza artificiale. Nuova Giur Civ Commentata Pt II:899–908
5. Cerea F (2024) Responsabilità civile e sistemi 'intelligenti'. Giappichelli, Torino
6. D'Adda A (2022) Danni 'da robot' (specie in ambito sanitario) e pluralità di responsabili tra sistema della responsabilità civile ed iniziative di diritto europeo. Riv Diritto Civ, 805–837
7. Di Donna L (2022) Intelligenza artificiale e rimedi risarcitori. Wolter Kluvers, Milano
8. D'Onofrio M (2024) Volontà e responsabilità dell'intelligenza artificiale: nuovi problemi e categorie tradizionali. In: La volontà macchinica. Pacini, Pisa, pp 17–42
9. Faccioli M (2024) La responsabilità civile per danni cagionati da sistemi di intelligenza artificiale nel prisma dell'onere della prova. Responsabilità civile e previdenza, 950–965
10. Finocchiaro G (2024) Intelligenza artificiale. Quali regole? Il Mulino, Bologna
11. Gentili A (2024) Regole per l'intelligenza artificiale. Contratto e impresa, 1043–1069
12. Lior A (2020) AI entities as AI agents: artificial intelligence liability and the AI *respondeat* superior analogy. Mitchell Hamline Law Rev, 1043–1102
13. Neuwirth RJ (2023) The EU artificial intelligence act. Regulating subliminal AI systems. Routledge, New York
14. Novelli C (2024) L'Artificial Intelligence Act Europeo: alcune questioni di implementazione. Federalismi, 95–113
15. Passagnoli G (2019) Ragionamento giuridico e tutele nell'intelligenza artificiale. Persona e mercato, 79–85
16. Pinelli C (2025) L'AI Act: gestione del rischio e tutela dei diritti. Giurispr Ital, 452–457
17. Proietti G (2024) Definire l'indefinibile? I sistemi di intelligenza artificiale alla ricerca di un inquadramento sistematico. Contratto e impresa, 882–925
18. Ratti M (2020) Riflessioni in materia di responsabilità civile e danno cagionato da dispositivo intelligente alla luce dell'attuale scenario normativo. Contratto e impresa, 1174–1191
19. Salanitro U (2020) Intelligenza artificiale e responsabilità: la strategia della commissione Europea. Riv Diritto Civ, 1246–1276
20. Sciarra MN (2020) La responsabilità delle macchine. Robotica e diritto dell'intelligenza artificiale. Pagine, Roma
21. Scognamiglio C (2023) Responsabilità civile ed intelligenza artificiale: quali soluzioni per quali problemi? Responsabilità civile e previdenza, 1073-1089
22. di Carlo MS (2024) La responsabilità connessa all'utilizzo dei sistemi di intelligenza artificiale. Danno Responsabilita, pp 421–429
23. Smorto G (2024) Distribuzione del rischio e tutela dei diritti nel regolamento europeo sull'intelligenza artificiale. Una riflessione critica. Foro Ital V:208–220
24. Zorzi Galgano N (2025) Il Regolamento UE 2024/1689 del 13 giugno 2024 sul c.d. alto rischio inaccettabile: le pratiche inerenti sistemi di intelligenza artificiale vietate dal legislatore europeo. Contratto e impresa, pp 45–94

Chapter 15
Closing Remarks

Stefano Campostrini

The richness of the presentations and contributions to this conference has been undeniably substantial. I would like to thank my colleagues who organized it, both for their efforts and for choosing such a relevant topic. In these final reflections, I will not attempt to summarize individual contributions—for obvious reasons of brevity and my own limitations—but instead offer some contextual elements to reinforce the importance of the subject and the challenges ahead. The various contributions have highlighted these challenges, and due to their scope, I believe no one aimed to solve them definitively.

As a good statistician, let me begin with some numbers. At the start of this millennium, in the Veneto region (where this conference is being held), there were just over 300,000 elderly people (according to the most recent legal definition, over 75 years old). About 365,000. Much of the socio-healthcare system was designed and planned around these figures. Today, that number has nearly doubled (well over 600,000), and the real challenge will emerge soon—in just over a decade—when the baby boomer generation will mostly be over 75. Forecasts indicate that in the 2040s, Veneto will count over one million residents aged over 75 [1].

These figures alone are staggering. But to grasp the full magnitude of the challenge facing our socio-healthcare systems [2], we need more context. The demographic transition we are experiencing is not just about the increase in life expectancy and the growing number of elderly and very elderly people. A parallel phenomenon—the sharp decline in birth rates—is significantly increasing the old-age dependency ratio. Without delving into details, consider this a few years ago, 500,000 elderly people "weighed" on a population of nearly five million in Veneto. The one million elderly forecast for 2040 will weigh on a population of just over four million.

S. Campostrini (✉)
Ca' Foscari University of Venice, Venice, Italy
e-mail: stefano.campostrini@unive.it

A. Bernes, S. Thobani (eds.), *Digitalisation in Health Care between New Technologies, Data and Research*, Services and Business Process Reengineering, https://doi.org/10.1007/978-981-95-6982-3_15

Another contextual consideration, relevant to the healthcare world, concerns the so-called epidemiological transition. Over the last century, we have moved from mortality (and morbidity) largely due to infectious diseases to over 80% of deaths and illnesses now being caused by non-communicable diseases (as defined by WHO)—which I prefer to call, using a term more common in healthcare, chronic diseases [3]. This term better reflects the fundamental difference between infectious and chronic diseases. For the former, healthcare intervention focuses on the acute phase, resolving the issue relatively quickly or, as in the past, the patient passed away rapidly. With chronic diseases, the onset marks the beginning of a long-term co-existence, often spanning decades, and typically involving multiple conditions (comorbidity). This has a clear impact both on the healthcare system's burden and the types of services required; and beyond hospital care, there is an increasing demand for community-based, health, and social-healthcare services.

Considering that these services are mostly needed in the advanced stages of chronic disease—usually beyond the age of 75—and combining this with the projected increase in the elderly population, we face a challenge of such magnitude that the current system of service provision cannot sustainably meet future demand. Individual demand is increasing, and so is the number of individuals with such needs.

I do not wish to add further gloomy notes to this scenario, which I dare to describe as a "perfect storm." (Please forgive my tone: I try to be as clear as possible, also terminologically, especially so that political and technical decision-makers realize the need to tackle these problems *hic et nunc*.) But there are more challenges: climate change, which already negatively impacts health; globalization, which—as we saw during the recent pandemic—removes borders for pathogens; migration, which presents both benefits (given demographic realities) to the society but also strains to healthcare systems.

Let me mention one last issue that, particularly in the Italian environment, contributes negatively to the perfect storm: the crisis in the healthcare workforce [4]. To the casual observer, this may appear as a crisis among doctors. But while some issues of planning and specialty imbalance exist there, the real crisis concerns nursing. In the context of healthcare's technological transformation, nursing is even more critical. We are now also seeing signs of strain in the lowest tier of the healthcare workforce hierarchy—social-healthcare workers—who are increasingly essential, especially in elderly care. Today, we seem to face a "vocational crisis" (though I argue this is misleading, since structural factors have made these professions less attractive, beyond simple spiritual or ethical considerations). Looking ahead, demographics are not in our favor: even if we succeed in making these jobs attractive again, the percentage of young people entering them will apply to a shrinking base. The cohort of young adults choosing careers in 2030–2040 will be nearly half the size it was in the early 2000s.

So, we complete the perfect storm scenario: rising demand and declining supply. The fundamental challenge for researchers and policymakers is thus to identify potential solutions.

The first option, in Italy, is to be rejected outright for constitutional reasons (thanks to the beautiful Article 32): offering full services only to some, while cutting back for others.

A second, more likely scenario is to lower the quality or breadth of services for everyone. Unfortunately, this is what we are already witnessing. In the absence of decisive reform, this path will be fully realized. In my view, this approach should also be rejected, as it fosters social tension (already detectable today) and deepens health inequalities. It may preserve formal adherence to the principles of equity and universal access (as enshrined in Article 32), but in substance, it undermines them.

In this perfect storm, the idea that new technologies might offer a panacea—a third solution—is incorrect or, at best, partial. For several reasons:

First (briefly, as it could get out of the scope of the present intervention) is the financial aspect. Technologies, especially when first introduced, often increase service costs. Efficiency gains (which alone cannot solve our challenges) only appear in the medium term and only if implementation is done correctly. Introducing technology en masse could initially worsen the healthcare system's financial sustainability.

Second is the organizational challenge. New technologies are useless without organizational changes. While technological innovation is already widespread in healthcare, organizational innovation is still in its infancy. There are successful examples where technological and organizational changes have been combined effectively—improving both impact and sustainability [5], but much has to be studied and implemented.

This leads to the third, and most relevant for this conference: the legal and regulatory dimension. It is inconceivable to implement technological and organizational innovations in a highly regulated system like healthcare without also changing its legal and regulatory framework.

In short, adopting more technology as an "exit strategy" without addressing these three aspects is like pouring new wine into old wineskins, as the Gospel warns.

If we do indeed need new wine—and I believe we do, urgently—we must also build new wineskins.

This is especially delicate in healthcare, which has a unique trait: it cannot stop to be fixed; it must change while in motion. As the pandemic showed, even short-term shutdowns carry enormous health and social costs. We must therefore maintain the old system temporarily, while experimenting with new models.

This has implications not only for systems (organizational and regulatory) but also for research. It has long been assumed that medical and technological research could run in parallel. Recently, it's become clear they must work together. The same now applies to organizational research: innovation in healthcare management must go hand-in-hand with technological, clinical, and procedural innovation.

After this contextual preamble, I believe the relevance of legal reflection is clearer. Legal norms are, in my view, an essential part of the healthcare system's organizational architecture. If this architecture must be fundamentally redesigned—as outlined above—legal contributions are key. A further challenge to my legal colleagues: in the past, law followed change. One experimented, consolidated, then regulated. Today, that sequence may no longer be viable. Given the magnitude and speed of change (in society, technology, and organization), law may need to accompany change, not follow it. Take this as a provocation from an outsider.

Finally, let me briefly reflect on some specific legal challenges that I see from my particular (and admittedly biased) perspective on healthcare systems. As a statistician, I have always dealt with data. Early in my career, I learned how closely data quality is tied to organizational structures. One early (unpublished) study of mine examined the quality of hospital records. It was poor. With the introduction of diagnosis-related groups—which linked those records to administrative and financial functions—data quality improved substantially, as did their use in epidemiological research. In short, data-regulation-organization forms an inseparable triad in healthcare.

This brings us to current technologies that could positively transform healthcare systems. Many hinge on data. Take the most disruptive innovation today: Artificial Intelligence. Despite its flashy name, AI is simply a highly advanced (not necessarily intelligent) use of large-scale data.

Success in healthcare AI (see [6, 7]) depends on how we handle the data-organization-regulation triad. AI is powerful, but also deeply invasive. Like any tool or procedure in healthcare, it must be tested, its organizational role defined, and it must be regulated.

But digitalization is not just AI. It includes the advanced use of digital tools to transform service delivery. One notable example is the virtual hospital [8], already operating in some areas. Through advanced technology and data—and a radically different organization—more patients can be treated at home, avoiding travel and hospital stays. This reduces costs for the system while improving patient experience. Is it technology? Of course. But what is truly striking is the organizational innovation. Nurses, for instance, remain the primary front line, but now serve many more patients. A brilliant way to optimize a scarce resource, as my economist colleagues would say.

Again, all this relies on sophisticated data use.

A final, slightly polemical but constructive note. If we agree that today's challenges demand disruptive approaches—in technology *and* organization—then legal frameworks must evolve as well. They too must adopt a disruptive mindset.

This is the challenge I leave to my legal colleagues (whose presentations here suggest they are more than capable). I confess some frustration (here comes the polemic) with the excessive restrictions on data use—especially for research—we face today, particularly in Europe, and even more so in Italy. Please don't misunderstand me: I fully support privacy and sensitive data protection. I simply believe we may be able to find alternatives to the default "it can't be done." Perhaps we need new wineskins for privacy and data use as well.

Bibliography

1. Bidoli C, Pegoraro V, Dal Mas F, Bagnoli C, Bert F, Bonin M, Butturini G, Cobianchi L, Cordiano C, Minto G, Pilerci C, Stocco P, Zantedeschi M, Campostrini S (2025) Virtual hospitals: the future of the healthcare system? An expert consensus. J Telemed Telecare 31(1):121–133
2. Cavazza A, Dal Mas F, Campostrini S, Biancone P, Degregori G, Brescia V (2025) The use of artificial intelligence in healthcare to promote sustainable development goals: a bibliometric review and a future research and policy agenda. In: EHMA 2025 taking action to improve health for all, European Health Management Association. EHMA, Convegno, pp 66–66
3. Harper S (2014) Economic and social implications of aging societies. Science 346(6209):587–591
4. JASON (2017) Artificial intelligence for health and health care. MITRE Corporation
5. Kickbusch I, Agrawal A, Jack A, Lee N, Horton R (2019) Governing health futures 2030: growing up in a digital world—a joint The Lancet and Financial Times Commission. Lancet 394(10206):1309
6. OECD (2021) Health at a glance 2021: OECD indicators. OECD Publishing
7. Rapporto statistico del Veneto (2024) https://statistica.regione.veneto.it/Pubblicazioni/RapportoStatistico2024/index.html
8. WHO (2015) World report on ageing and health. World Health Organization

FSC
www.fsc.org
MIX
Papier | Fördert
gute Waldnutzung
FSC® C083411

Kolibri 360 GmbH
Ferdinand-Jühlke-Straße 7
99095 Erfurt, Deutschland
produktsicherheit@kolibri360.de